Atlas of Microscopic Artifacts and Foreign Materials

Atlas of Microscopic Artifacts and Foreign Materials

I-Tien Yeh, M.D.
Pathologist
Abington Memorial Hospital
Abington, PA

John S. J. Brooks, M.D. MRCPath
Chairman & Professor of Pathology
Roswell Park Cancer Institute
Buffalo, NY

Giuseppe G. Pietra, M.D.
Professor Emeritus
University of Pennsylvania Medical Center
Philadelphia, PA

Editor: Charles W. Mitchell
Marketing Manager: Lorraine A. Smith
Production Coordinator: Dana M. Soares
Typesetter: Better Graphics, Inc.
Printer: Quebacor Printing Book Group

351 West Camden Street
Baltimore, Maryland 21201-2436 USA

Rose Tree Corporate Center
1400 North Providence Road
Building II, Suite 5025
Media, Pennsylvania 19063-2043 USA

Accurate indications, adverse reactions and dosage schedules for drugs are provided in this book, but is it possible that they may change. The reader is urged to review the package information data of the manufacturers of the medications mentioned.

Printed in the United States of America

First Edition,

Library of Congress Cataloging-in-Publication Data

RB43 . Y44 1997
Atlas of microscopic artifacts and foreign materials / I-Tien Yeh;
with contributions from John S. J. Brooks, Giuseppe G. Pietra.
p. cm.
Includes bibliographical references and index.
1. Medical microscopy—Atlases. I. Brooks, John S. J.
II. Pietra, Giuseppe G. III. Title
[DNLM: 1. Microscopy—atlases. 2. Histology—atlases.
3. Artifacts—atlases. QS 517 Y43a 1997]
616.07′58—dc21
DNLM/DLC
for Library of Congress 96-50067
CIP

ISBN: 0-683-30332-5

The publishers have made every effort to trace the copyright holders for borrowed material. If they have inadvertently overlooked any, they will be pleased to make the necessary arrangements at the first opportunity.

To purchase additional copies of this book, call our customer service department at **(800) 638-0672** or fax orders to **(800) 447-8438**. For other book services, including chapter reprints and large quantity sales, ask for the Special Sales department.

Canadian customers should call **(800) 665-1148**, or fax **(800) 665-0103**. For all other calls originating outside of the United States, please call **(410) 528-4233** or fax us at **(410) 528-8550**.

Visit Williams & Wilkins on the Internet: **http://www.wwilkins.com** or contact our customer service department at **custserv@wwilkins.com**. Williams & Wilkins customer service representatives are available from 8:30 am to 6:00 pm, EST, Monday through Friday, for telephone access.

96 97 98 99 00
1 2 3 4 5 6 7 8 9 10

Preface

AN APPROACH TO MICROSCOPIC ARTIFACTS AND FOREIGN MATERIALS

An artifact may be defined as a structure or substance not normally present, but produced by some external agency or action. In the examination of pathologic specimens in a routine hospital practice, we come across many tissue substances that are the result of disease processes, such as cystine crystals due to congenital metabolic disease. Strictly speaking, these crystals are not artifacts, since they are not produced by an external process, but by a disease process that allows the excess accumulation of cystine. Nevertheless, the crystals are not normally present and are considered in this book, since they are in the differential diagnosis of true artifacts. External agents, such as dusts, may be inhaled, ingested, or introduced by trauma. Other artifacts are produced as the result of medical intervention or handling of the specimen after receipt in the laboratory. In this monograph, we attempt to illustrate and aid in the identification of some of the more common artifacts and foreign materials that are found in tissue specimens.

Similar to any diagnostic workup, the explanation of the source of the artifact often lies with the patient's medical history and in communication with our clinical colleagues. Retracing the steps that the specimen has taken, from gross room handling, to the processing and staining of the specimen, will resolve many of the remainder of the mysteries.

Identification of large objects may be obvious on careful gross examination. Specimen radiographs can be performed if necessary. For small objects, light microscopy is sufficient for the identification of many common artifacts.

The pattern and location of the artifact should be noted. An artifact present only at the edge of the tissue may be due to surgical handling or laboratory processing. A uniform process suggests an intrinsic process. An intracellular deposit often has different implications from an extracellular deposit. Many intracellular deposits are specific for a cell type, such as Russell bodies in plasma cells. Extracellular deposits may also depend upon the particular type of cells that produced the material, such as psammoma body formation from glandular cells. The plane of focus of the artifact should be compared with the plane of focus of the remainder of the tissue. Foreign materials are often seen in a different plane, because they tend to fracture when sectioned and often do not adhere well to glass slides. The microtome knife may even transport the material to a site distant from the original lodging place of the material. Tissue crevices may contain cells dragged there by a knife blade during sectioning ("knife metastasis").

The presence or absence of a tissue reaction is important to note. The presence of a tissue reaction implies that foreign material is truly embedded into the tissue and that sufficient time has ensued for the tissue reaction to occur. The cell types in the reactive process may be helpful in the identification of specific foreign materials, since materials will often elicit similar responses from patient to patient, and different materials will elicit different responses. The pattern of reaction can be assessed to predict the length of time the material has been in place. Although tissue reaction to foreign material is usually an inflammatory response, other events may occur, such as thrombogenesis, potentiation of infection, and even carcinogenesis. The absence of a reaction may indicate that the material is nonantigenic or that it is simply a normal component of the tissue. Alternatively, the lack of response may indicate that the artifact was introduced after the tissue was removed from the patient.

Cellular material may not necessarily be human. Clues to plant origin include a cellulose cell wall, presence of plastids, and starch grains. Insects and worms contain chitin cuticles.

The color, shape, and size of the material will aid greatly in its identification. The chapter on pigmented deposits will explore the color issue in more depth. The shape and size of the material are dictated by a variety of factors, and may be characteristic of the material in question.

Polarization light microscopy is easily performed. Many foreign materials are birefringent. Some materials are more easily seen with polarized light. When viewed with crossed polarizing filters, *anistropic* substances have the ability to separate light waves into two rays and will appear bright in a dark background. Substances that do not polarize are called *isotropic.*

Occasionally, necrotic tissue is removed and requires identification. Typically, malignant tumors outgrow their blood supply and central portions necrotize. At times, the biopsied necrotic tissue is all that is available. Close examination of the ghost outlines of cellular architecture is important, paying attention to cell size and shape, overall cellularity, and nuclear outlines. Immunohistochemical and other special stains can still be utilized to determine cellular differentiation characteristics.

To summarize, this simple procedure may be followed when confronted with an unknown material or possible artifact:

1) Check clinical history.
2) Review gross examination and tissue processing procedures.
3) Microscopic examination
   a) Focus up and down to determine the focal plane.
   b) Note tissue type and any tissue reaction.
   c) Note color, size, and shape and compare to known objects.
   d) Try to polarize the material.

If this procedure fails to adequately identify the artifact in question, special stains or other techniques may be required to study materials. The repertoire of special stains is large and other venerable monographs detail the procedures. The material may even need to be extracted from the tissue block for definitive identification. Hard materials, such as metals and ceramics, may need methacrylate embedding and grinding. Scanning electron microscopy will demonstrate surface characteristics, whereas transmission electron microscopy will provide further magnification (or in the words of one of my teachers, it will make what you don't know bigger!). Electron probe x-ray analysis (also known as energy dispersive x-ray analysis, EDX) is a nondestructive technique that can give in situ identification of minerals and metals. Although not routinely available in community hospital laboratories, these techniques may occasionally be necessary for medical–legal applications.

This book shall concentrate on routinely available stains and techniques in the hospital histology laboratory.

I-Tien Yeh, M.D.

DEDICATION

To my husband and best friend, Richard J. Lamb
and to my children, Jade and Jonathan

Acknowledgments

The photographs in this book have been made possible by many who have contributed support, glass slides, and expertise, including my colleagues at Abington Memorial Hospital, Drs. Herbert E. Auerbach, Paul J. Cherney, Richard T. Goldhahn, and Salvatore M. Valenti. Residents in the pathology department at the University of Pennsylvania helped collect some of the glass slides. The histologic preparations were often difficult to cut and consisted of extra blocks on top of a heavy load, but were provided with cheerfulness (usually!) by Deena Devine, Cheryl McMullen, Marie Duke Murphy, and Donna Suermann. Marleen Adams, Sharon Atkins, Joan Gregorio, Tina Harple, and Cathy Hildebrand provided the necessary office assistance, likewise on top of busy schedules.

Contributors

John S. J. Brooks, M.D., MRCPath
Chairman and Professor of Pathology
Roswell Park Cancer Institute
Buffalo, New York

Giuseppe G. Pietra, M.D.
Professor Emeritus
University of Pennsylvania Medical Center
Philadelphia, Pennsylvania

Contents

1

Artifacts of Fixation and Processing

Between the time a specimen is removed from a patient and a microscopic slide is created, there are numerous opportunities to introduce artifacts into the tissue. These include improper tissue preservation, freezing of tissue, and processing artifacts caused by the way tissue is placed into cassettes, as well as sectioning and coverslipping problems. These artifacts can and do occur with any type of tissue.

LACK OF PROPER PRESERVATION

Tissue may be either inadequately fixed or overfixed. Of the two problems, inadequate fixation is by far the most common. Tissue that has not been properly fixed tends to be soft and mottled in color, typically with the central portion appearing the same color as in the fresh state. Causes of inadequate fixation include lack of tissue exposure to fixative, prolonged time prior to placement of specimen into fixative, inadequate fixative to specimen ratio, and insufficient time for fixation.

The total lack of fixative or any liquid may occur at any point prior to paraffin: specimens may be left in the clinician's office or operating room without fixation; specimens may be forgotten in an obscure location; a small specimen may cling to the side of a container above the liquid/air interface; specimens may be left out on the surgical bench; the tissue processor may malfunction during a dry period. The list goes on and on—after a few years in pathology, most of us have our own war stories to tell. Prolonged periods without liquid typically leaves the specimens desiccated. Gross signs of desiccation include shrinkage and hardening of tissue. After extended desiccation, tissue is not easily rehydrated and the hardening may cause difficulty in cutting the blocks. Microscopically, there is poor cellular detail; the nuclei appear shrunken, and chromatin is smudged. Conversely, interstitial spaces are expanded. Rehydration may be attempted by placing the specimen in fixative. The paraffin block may be partially rehydrated with a piece of wet, lukewarm cotton followed by an ice cube.

Although we are classically taught that adequate fixation occurs only if the ratio of fixative to tissue is greater that 10 to 1, the reality of today's surgical pathology laboratory is that for large specimens, this ratio is often impossible to achieve. The reasons for this are multiple: the clinician is not aware of this ideal ratio and sends a 500-gm specimen down to pathology in 10 cc of fixative; some specimens are so large that no containers are available in the laboratory that would fulfill this ratio; the costs of formalin and its disposal (or of alternative fixatives) are high and minimization of use of fixative is encouraged by cost containment guidelines of hospitals. Tissue may be in a container with fixative and still not be adequately fixed. If a specimen is not opened or sliced so that the maximal thickness of tissue is less than 1 cm, the time required for penetration of the specimen by fixative will be excessive, and specimen degradation will occur. Specimen degradation typically presents as autolysis, as commonly seen in autopsy tissue, due to enzymatic digestion. In this process, cells are dissociated and tissue dissolution takes place. Solutions to these problems include immediate opening and fixation, extending the fixation time, increasing the ratio of fixative used, and decreasing the thickness of cut tissue.

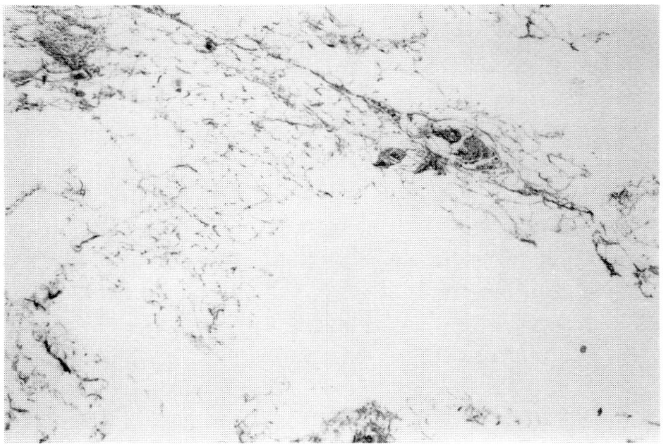

Fig. 1.1. Poor fixation, breast biopsy. This specimen was largely composed of adipose tissue, which fixes slowly. The edges of the specimen were better fixed than central portions. Inadequately fixed areas were too soft to be cut properly on the microtome, thus leaving big gaps in the tissue.

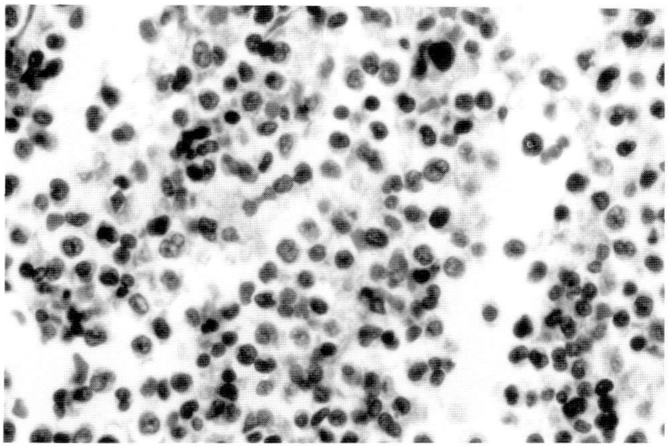

Fig. 1.2. Autolysis, bone marrow. This specimen was from a patient with acute myelocytic leukemia, at autopsy. Individual cells are separated from one another due to partial lysis.

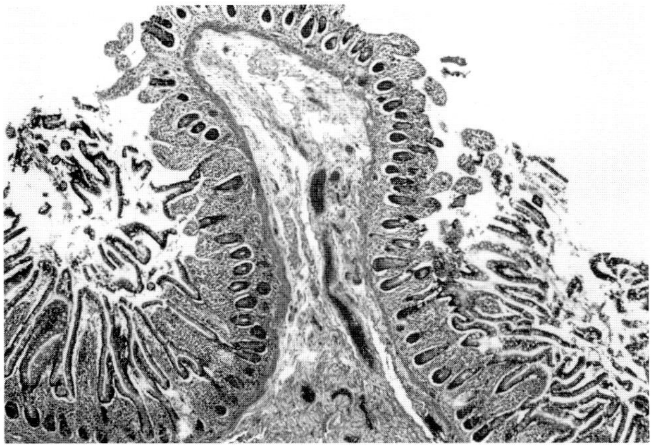

Fig. 1.3. Autolysis, small bowel. This bowel had been placed into a container without fixative for several hours. Epithelial cells become detached from each other and from the underlying stroma.

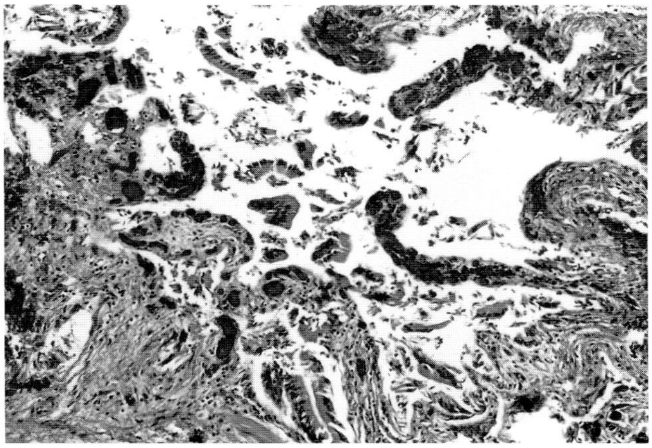

Fig. 1.4. Autolysis, gallbladder. The gallbladder was removed intact and placed into fixative. However, it was full of bile for several hours prior to sectioning by the pathologist. The epithelium is completely lysed, and only the epithelial cells within crypts can be seen.

Tissue is sometimes not fixed by the clinician prior to receipt by pathology. Receipt of a fresh specimen is necessary if special studies need to be performed on the tissue other than the usual processing. If tissue is put in an isotonic solution of saline, no significant changes in cellular morphology should occur. Nevertheless, several problems may arise. If the tissue remains at room temperature without fixation for a prolonged period of time, bacterial overgrowth may occur, particularly with contaminated specimens such as bowels and placentas, which tend to be removed at night or weekends and left in the operating room or on pathology's counter instead of the refrigerator. We have even had a couple of placentas placed in our histology lab's oven by inattentive night staff. The stench of the specimen is a good clue of the bacterial contamination when you open the container. Microscopically, either pure colonies or mixed colonies of bacteria will be seen, usually heaviest at the edges of the specimen and without significant host response (i.e., no leukocytes in the vicinity). These colonies are usually easily seen on the hematoxylin–eosin (H&E) stain as a fuzzy blue rim around tissue on low power, and as small rod or coccal-shaped organisms on higher power. Tissue breakdown occurs with heavy bacterial contamination.

Refrigeration of specimens will delay the process of autolysis and is preferable in instances when fixation cannot be accomplished immediately. However, lack of fixation does lead to tissue dehydration, as noted above.

Solutions to these problems lie with educating the clinicians to properly fix specimens and/or transport the specimens to the laboratory promptly, as well as having a workable regimen for notification of the laboratory that a specimen has been sent. Overnight refrigeration is an option if necessary.

Conversely, overfixation may occur. Prolonged exposure to formalin may cause excessive cross-linkage and difficulty in staining tissue antigens by immunohistochemistry. On H&E stain, there is increased tissue shrinkage, but usually no significant staining differences are seen if buffered formalin is used. Years of tissue storage in formalin may cause decreased stain intake. Prolonged fixation in mercuric chloride based fixatives, such as Zenker's, will cause acidophilia. Mercuric chloride crystals may form. Use of a sodium bicarbonate solution prior to H&E staining will solve this problem. With Bouin's fixation, incomplete removal of picric acid from the tissue blocks can cause tissue degradation with time. The sooner sections are cut from the block, the better the preservation of tissue will appear.

Tissue in hypotonic solutions, such as distilled water prior to processing, will show hydropic degenerative changes. In skin specimens, bullous lesions may occur which are difficult to distinguish from in situ changes.

Ethanol fixation causes dehydration, which in turn causes cellular shrinkage. Red blood cells are lysed. Staining characteristics with special stains may also be altered.

FREEZING

Frozen sections are utilized for microscopic examinations during an intraoperative consultation, for immunohistochemical staining for some antigens, and for confirmation of tissue histology before performance of further laboratory tests, such as estrogen receptor assays.

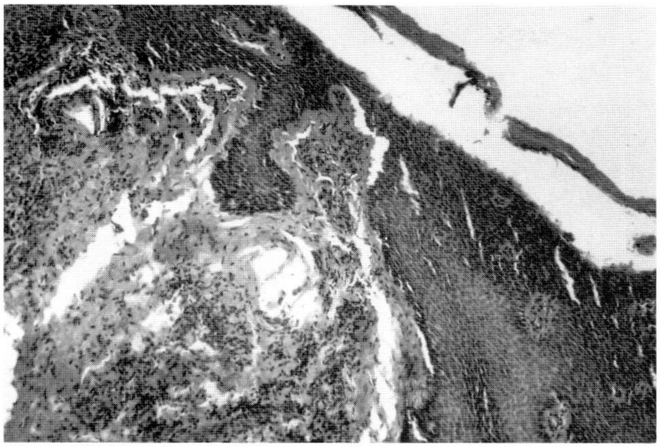

Fig. 1.5. Drying artifact, vulva. This vulvar biopsy was inadvertently left out overnight in a cassette, without any fluid. The edges of the tissue are dark and shrunken. The dried tissue is difficult to cut, and cracking artifact is present. Cellular areas away from the edge appear lighter, more spread out.

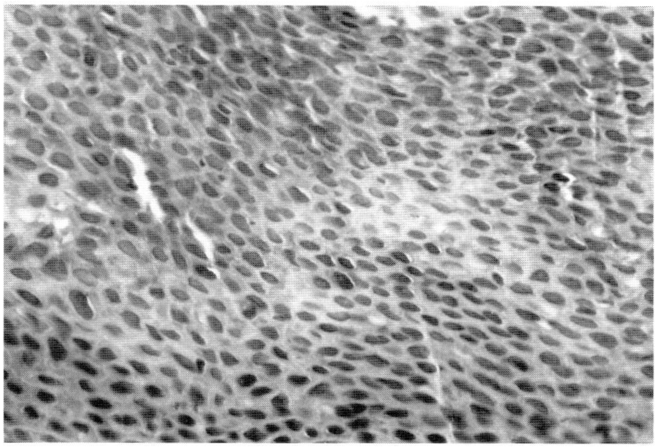

Fig. 1.6. Dried specimen, high power. Nuclear detail is lost.

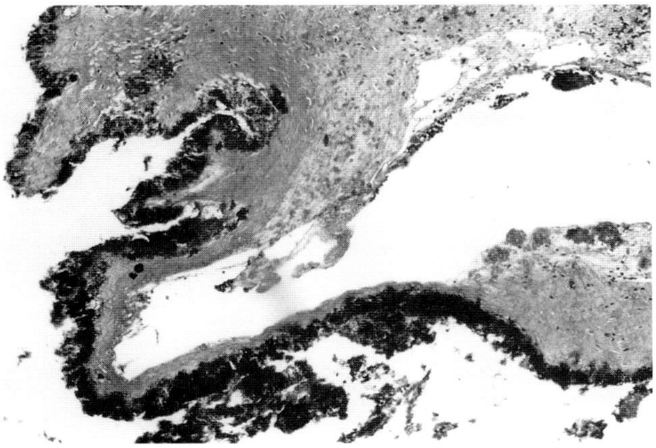

Fig. 1.7. Bacterial proliferation, colon. The low-power micrograph demonstrates a linear dark area at the serosal surface of a ruptured diverticulum.

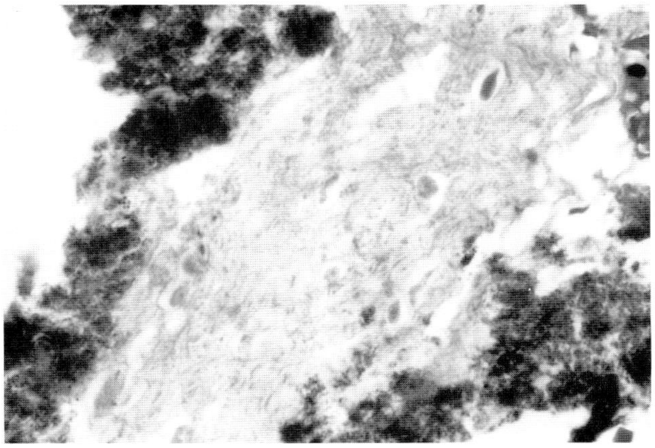

Fig. 1.8. Bacterial proliferation, colon. Higher power of the dark area reveals numerous coccal bacteria in this dark area.

When tissue is frozen, it becomes dehydrated; ice crystals form both intra- and extracellularly. After the frozen sections are cut, tissue is usually thawed by placement into a fixative. Disrupted or collapsed cells result from melting of the ice. Cells often look shrunken and interstitium is expanded with artifactural spaces. Nuclei can be displaced, forming signet ring like cells, due to the vacuolization of the cytoplasm. Tissues with relatively low water content, such as fibrous tissue, withstand freezing better than those with high water content, such as kidney biopsies. Adipose tissue is difficult to freeze; the fat provides insulation and slows the speed of freezing.

Once ice crystals have formed, there is no ready solution to this artifact. Prevention is the best tactic. Minimizing this artifact includes freezing the tissue as quickly as possible; the faster the freezing process, the smaller the ice crystals formed. Freezing that occurs in a liquid with a low freezing point, such as liquid nitrogen, accomplishes freezing faster than low temperature air in a cryostat. Use of fluorinated hydrocarbons to quick freeze specimens can leave oil-like residue or cause dehydration/cracking of tissue. In addition, the smaller the piece of tissue, the more quickly the specimen will freeze. Avoid the freezing of adipose tissue, which cuts poorly and insulates the remainder of the tissue. Therefore, a small piece of tissue, relatively uninsulated, placed in liquid freezing media, will show the least artifact.

BONE DUST

The cutting of bone, either by the surgeon or the pathologist, may produce dust-like particles of bone. Grossly, bone dust appears as wet sawdust and is typically present at the cut surface of bone. This material may be pushed into marrow spaces and sometimes contains air bubbles. Microscopically, bone dust is composed of irregular eosinophilic particles of varying sizes. It can be differentiated from a fracture site by the lack of accompanying hemorrhage or cellular reaction. The artifact is less when manual tools are used, as opposed to powered saws. Sampling of tissue away from the sites of saw cuts will also avoid this artifact.

SPONGE ARTIFACT

Bristles from polyfoam sponges, used to hold small fragments of tissue in processing cassettes, have been implicated in causing artifacts in tissue sections. The typical appearance is of angulated defects within tissue, with discrete edges and smooth contours. Often, the cells at the edge of the defect are flattened and may resemble endothelial cells. The degree of artifact is related to the consistency of the tissue; that is, the softer the tissue, the more likely it is to be compressed by the bristles. Firmer tissues, with more supporting matrix and vasculature, will show the least amount of damage. To avoid this artifact, use alternate means of securing small tissue fragments in cassettes for soft specimens such as brain, where the distortion may hamper the diagnosis.

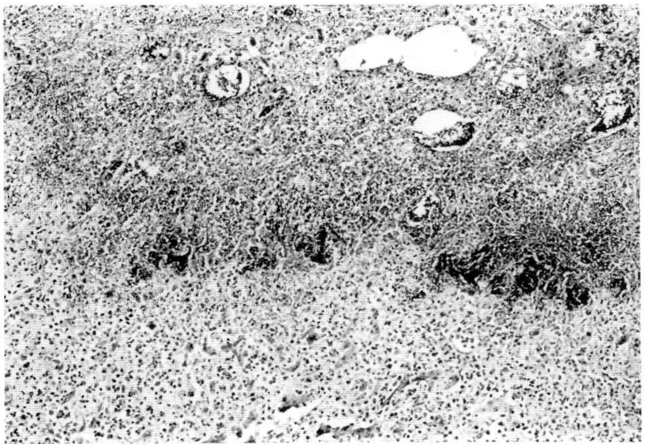

Fig. 1.9. Bacterial proliferation, liver. This liver was from an autopsy case in which the patient's body had remained at room temperature for many hours prior to examination. A linear dark area is present.

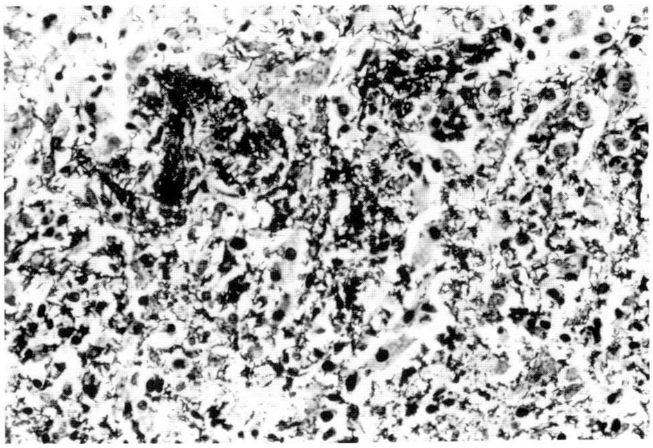

Fig. 1.10. Bacterial proliferation, liver. Hepatocytes are separated from one another by numerous rod-shaped bacteria. Note lack of cellular reaction.

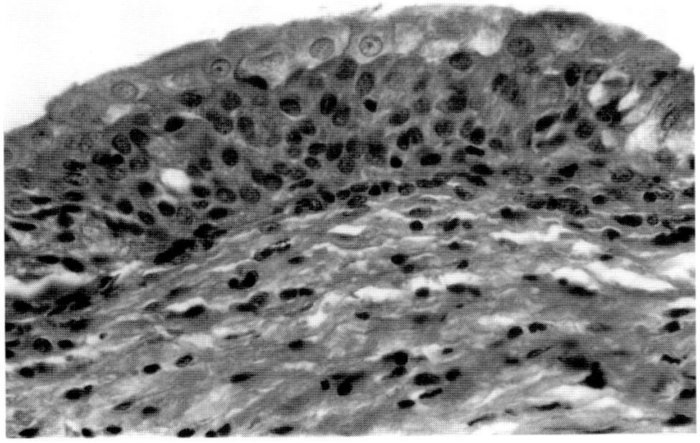

Fig. 1.11. Hydropic change, bladder biopsy. Distilled water had been used to rinse the bladder. The surface umbrella cells of the transitional epithelium are swollen due to the hypotonic fluid.

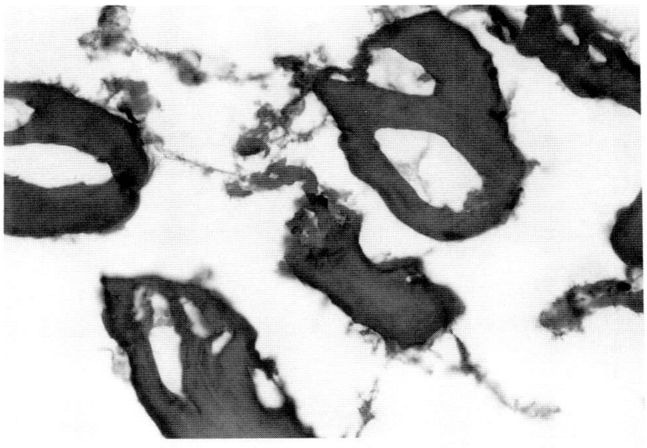

Fig. 1.12. Freezing artifact, skeletal muscle. The muscle fibers show distortion by the formation of ice crystals within fibers.

PIGMENTED GRANULES

Probably the most common problem with granules formed during fixation is the so-called "formalin pigment." Formalin pigment appears as anisotropic black granules in bloody formalin-fixed tissues. It forms as the result of a reaction between formic acid of unbuffered formalin with the heme of hemoglobin. Formalin pigment may be removed by a variety of organic and inorganic methods. Prevention of this artifact is through the use of buffered, rather than acid, formalin.

Dark brown granules may be seen in Bouin's fixed tissues when decreased proportions of picric or acetic acid or both, are used.

Basophilic deposits of calcium in interstitium may be caused by calcium acetate or calcium carbonate used as neutralizing agents in buffered formalin. Stains for calcium will be positive. Mucopolysaccharide staining may distinguish calcium precipitant form tissue calcium, since true calcification is typically associated with mucopolysaccharides and pseudocalcification is not.

SECTIONING ARTIFACTS

Several types of artifacts may be produced at the time of sectioning the paraffin block on the microtome. The classical **"Venetian blind"** effect is described as lengthwise scratch marks. These marks are caused by vibrations while sectioning, either because of a loose microtome knife, contamination of the knife edge, or differences in the hardness of the tissue within the block. A clean knife, properly fastened, may solve the problem. If the cause is the block, then soaking the block prior to sectioning may lessen the effect of alternate tissue hardness.

Dull knives may cause tissue compression and "chatter". **Compression** occurs when the knife is at an extreme angle to the tissue. If only a portion of the knife is dull, a linear streak in the section will be seen. If the entire knife is dull, the compression effect will be diffuse. At times, a dull knife may push fragments of tissue over, so that the fragments overlay other tissue pieces. **Chatter** is described as alternating thick and thin zones in tissue sections, and can be caused by knife dullness or vibrations from a loose knife or unstable specimen chuck. Sharpening the knife blade, changing the knife, or stabilizing the specimen will solve these problems.

If small amounts of processing or clearing fluids remain in the block after embedding, **wrinkled sections** may result. When incompletely cleared tissue sections are placed in the water bath, they do not expand in proportion to the amount of water taken in. Conversely, inadequate dehydration of tissue will prevent adequate penetration of tissue by wax. Incomplete paraffinization makes the tissue difficult to cut. Reprocessing the tissue may be attempted to correct these effects.

CONTAMINANTS

Various contaminants may be present at any point in the processing sequence. During surgery, tissue may be carried from one site to another, especially loosely cohesive fragments of tumor. Recently, a newly described cardiovas-

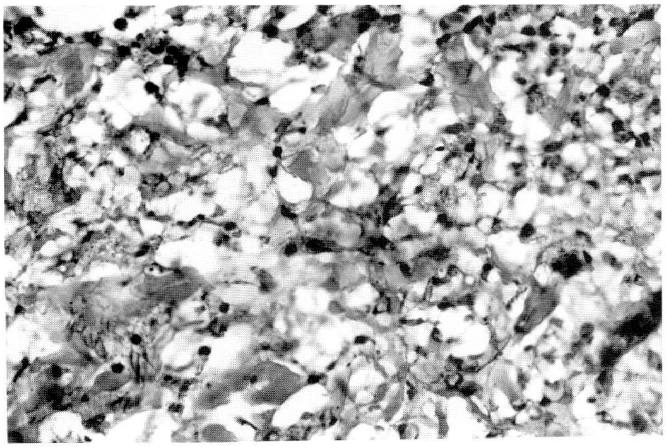

Fig. 1.13. Freezing artifact, lymph node. Intracellular ice disrupts cell membranes and extracellular ice pushes cells into abnormal formations. Many of the lymphocytes artifactually appear to be signet ring cells due to ice crystals.

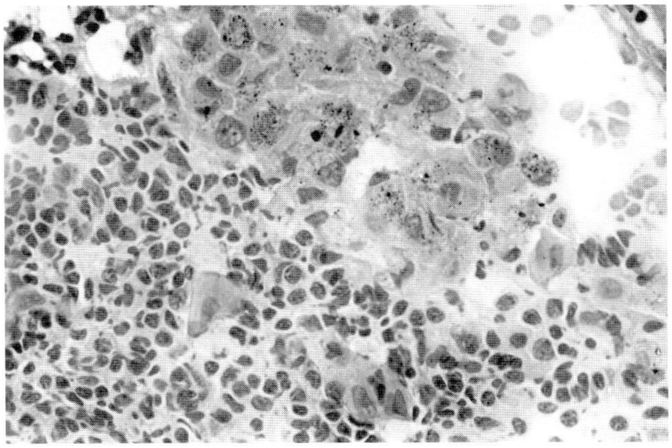

Fig. 1.14. Drying artifact, frozen section of lymph node. If a frozen section is not immediately fixed, air drying of the section takes place. The cells appear larger than normal, with blown up nuclei, particularly at tissue edges (*upper right corner photograph*).

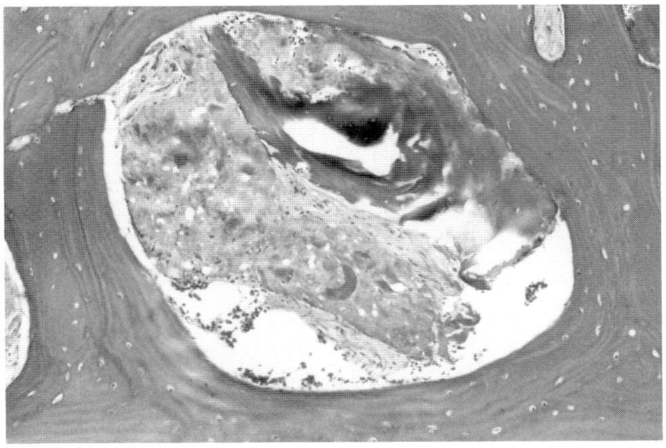

Fig. 1.15. Bone dust. The mechanical effect of the saw on bone fragments it into tiny particles, usually seen at the edge of the specimen near the point of sawcut. The material appears as eosinophilic fragments, often with air bubbles, which may be pushed into a preexisting space.

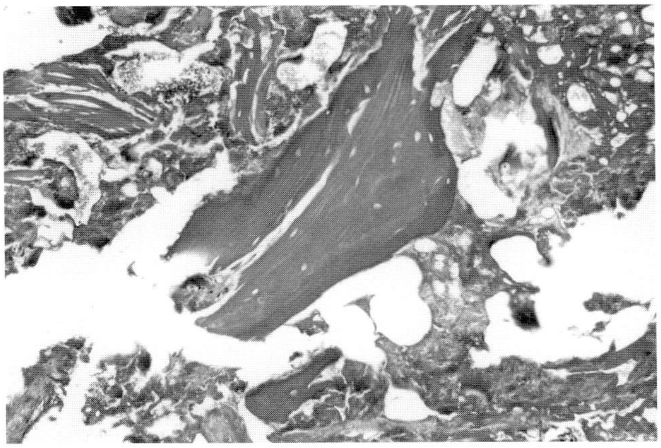

Fig. 1.16. Bone dust, high power. Irregularly shaped bone particles, pushed together and with clear round air bubbles.

cular lesion was shown to be an artifact of cardiotomy suction. The most common contaminants include tissue carryover from the knife blade, cutting board, water bath, or any of the fluid media. Bacteria may grow in the water or gelatin and be seen on tissue sections. Particulate material may precipitate from stains to coat the slides. Most of the time, these problems are easily detectable because the tissue in question is obviously different from the remainder of the specimen and appears to be fragmented. Contaminant organisms and precipitants evoke no tissue response and are frequently seen at a different plane of focus.

Other examples of contaminants include: black material from pencil graphite or cigarette ashes (no longer a problem in smoke-free hospitals), lint fibers from clothing or gauze, and squames shed from the skin of histotechnologists.

MOUNTING ARTIFACTS

The temperature of waterbath is crucial to correct mounting. The water must be warm enough to spread tissue out, but not too hot or there will be overexpansion of tissue sections. Tissue will then shrink upon drying and slide adhesion is poor.

If there is air under a section when it is picked up on glass, the tissue on top shatters when the air bubble breaks. The tissue stains more intensely because tissue is exposed on two sides to solutions (both over and under the tissue).

Drying of a section at room temperature prior to staining may cause an erratic staining pattern.

COVERSLIPPING ARTIFACTS

During the process of coverslipping, there may be either too much or too little mounting media or adhesive. Excessive adhesives present as basophilic or acidophilic strands or splotches. Under the microscope, the sections may appear hazy. The edges of the slides are frequently sticky and may have beads of adhesive on top of the coverslip. Removing the coverslip and remounting will cure this problem. Otherwise, the mounting media may be too viscous and need to be thinned.

More frequently, air bubbles form. More numerous problems with air bubbles are seen using a coverslipping machine because the mounting media must be relatively thin for the machine to work. The sections are usually fine for a day or two after mounting, but when the xylene evaporates, air bubbles appear. Decreasing the amount of xylene in the mounting media is usually necessary. Too little xylene can also cause air bubbles by trapping air underneath mounting media. In cytologic specimens, air may be trapped under individual cells, giving the cells a golden, slightly raised appearance, known as "cornflaking" because of its microscopic resemblance to the breakfast cereal.

The coverslip should be an appropriate size for the tissue. Fading will occur peripherally if the tissue is too close to the edge, i.e., the coverslip is too small for the tissue. This effect usually appears some weeks after coverslipping. An oversized coverslip is usually not a problem, except that if the tissue is very small, it may be difficult to identify where it is on the slide.

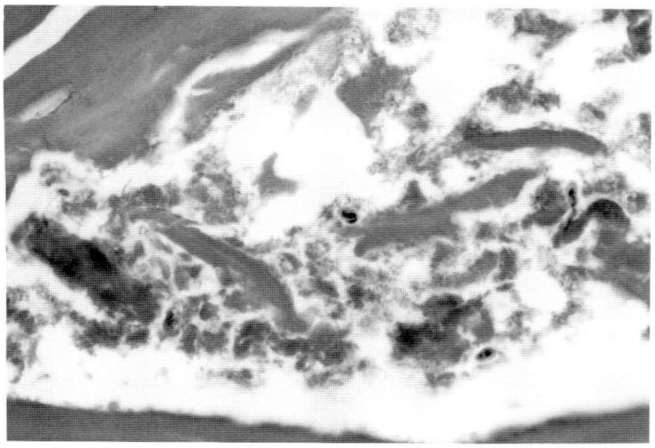

Fig. 1.17. Bone dust. Small irregular fragments of bone, with granular eosinophilic dusty bone pieces, are present at the edge of bone that has been cut with an electric saw.

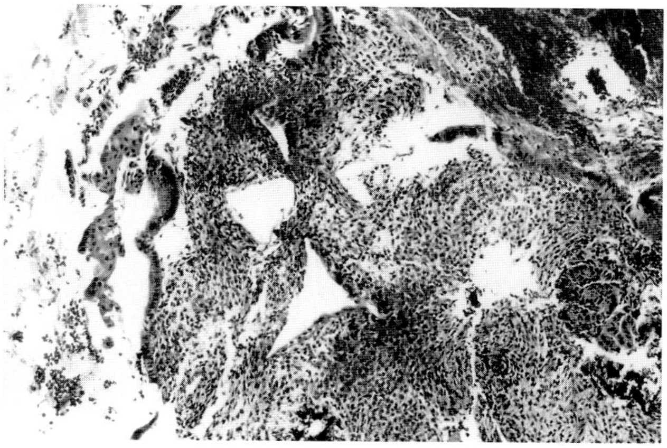

Fig. 1.18. Sponge artifact, endometrial biopsy. This artifact is produced during processing of soft biopsies in polyfoam sponges. Angulated spaces are present.

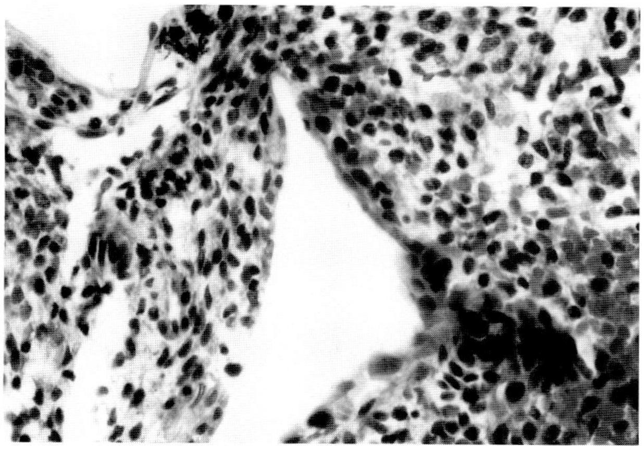

Fig. 1.19. Sponge artifact, endometrial biopsy. At high power, some of the spaces resemble distorted glandular or vascular spaces.

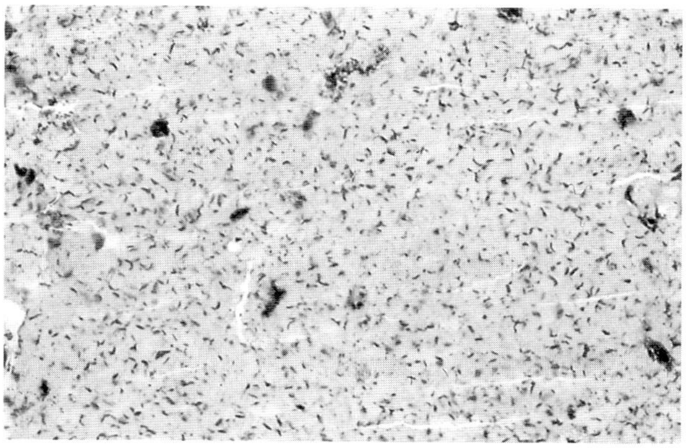

Fig. 1.20. Formalin pigment, hemorrhagic lung. Numerous uniformly sized refractile brown granules are present within the blood.

BIBLIOGRAPHY

Courtice RW, Stinson WA, Walley VM: Tissue fragments recovered at cardiac surgery masquerading as tumoral proliferations. *Am J Surg Pathol* 18:167–174, 1994.

Drury RAB, Wallington EA: *Carlton's Histological Technique*. Oxford, Oxford University Press, 1980.

Johnson FB: Identification of graphite in tissue sections. *Arch Pathol Lab Med* 104:491–492, 1980.

Landas SK, Bromley CM: Sponge artifact in biopsy specimens. *Arch Pathol Lab Med* 114:1285–1287, 1990.

Luna LG: *Histopathologic Methods and Color Atlas of Special Stains and Tissue Artifacts*. Gaithersburg, MD, American Histolabs, Inc, 1992.

Luna LG: Method for reprocessing dried tissue specimens. *Histo-Logic* 8:111, 1978.

Luthringer DJ, Virmani BG, Weiss SW, et al: A distinctive cardiovascular lesion resembling histiocytoid (epithelioid) hemangioma: evidence suggesting mesothelial participation. *Am J Surg Pathol* 14:993–1000, 1990.

Sheehan DC, Hrapchak BB: *Theory and Practice of Histotechnology*, ed 2. St Louis, CV Mosby, 1980.

Youngson BJ, Liberman L, Rosen PP: Displacement of carcinomatous epithelium in surgical breast specimens following stereotaxic core biopsy. *Am J Clin Pathol* 103:598–602, 1995.

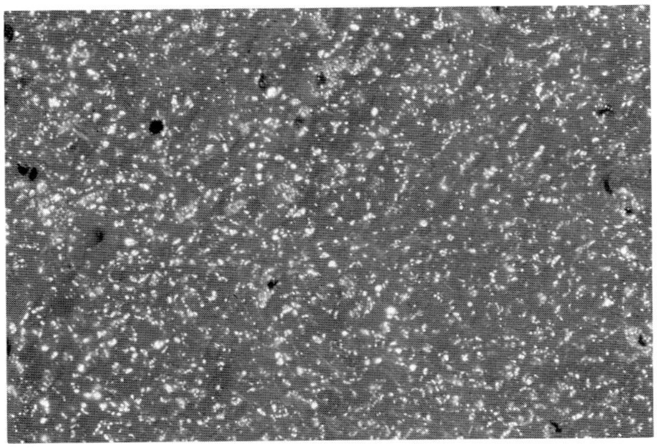

Fig. 1.21. Formalin pigment, hemorrhagic lung, polarized light microscopy. Polarization light microscopy will bring out formalin pigment (hematin), but not hemosiderin.

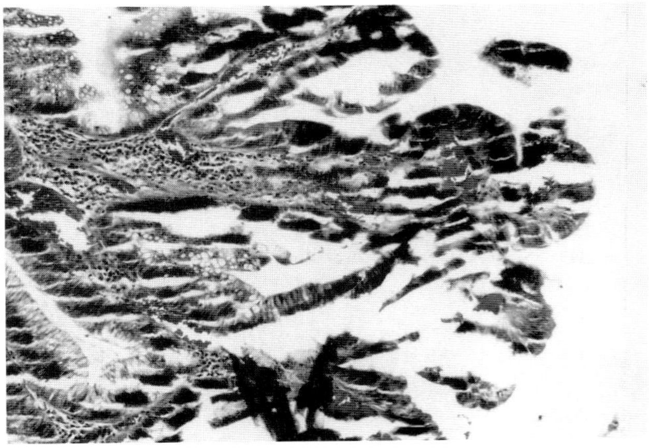

Fig. 1.22. Colon biopsy with "venetian blind" artifact. Note parallel lines of compressed tissue, alternating with open spaces. This artifact can be produced by vibration of the microtome knife, a loose block during sectioning, or tissue that has been overdehydrated in the block.

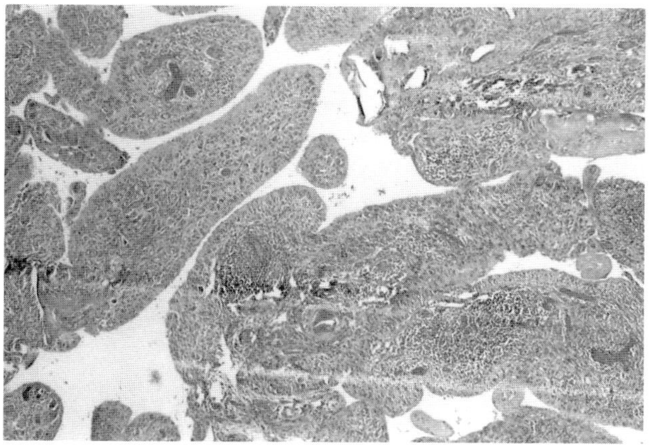

Fig. 1.23. Compression knife marks. Parallel streaks in tissue sections, with thinner area (*upper streak*) and small irregular tears in the tissue (*lower streaks*).

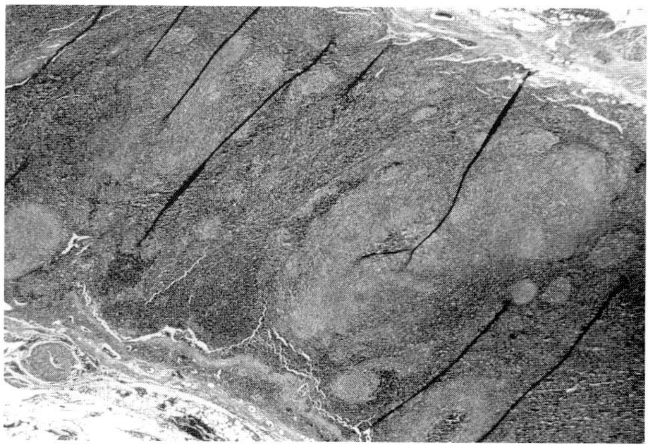

Fig. 1.24. Compression and folding, lymph node. Multiple tissue folds are noted, in parallel arrangement.

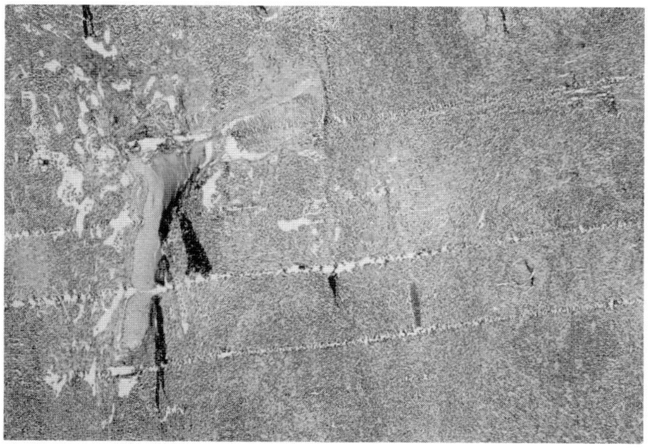

Fig. 1.25. Knife marks. There were nicks in the cutting edge of the knife. Linear streaks across the entire tissue section are seen. Note darkened edges next to clear zones, where cells have been pushed onto adjacent areas.

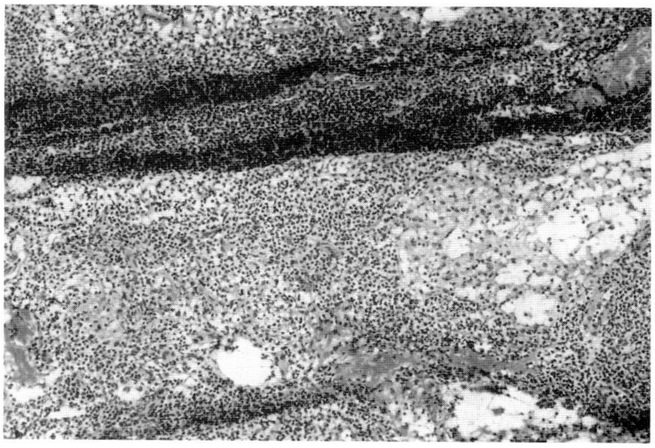

Fig. 1.26. Tissue fold. The dark area represents more than one layer of tissue. Cells are difficult to focus in this area.

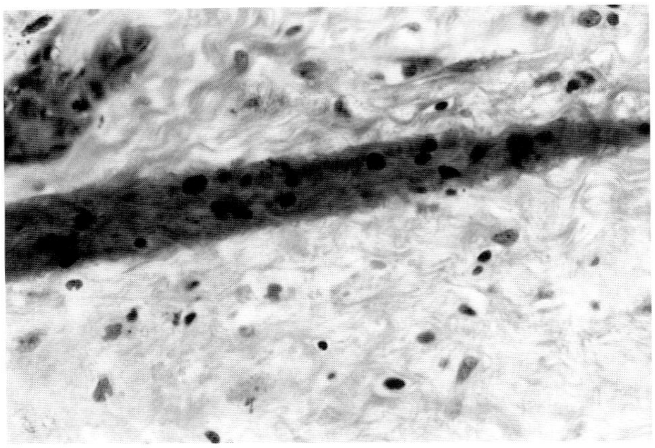

Fig. 1.27. Folded tissue. The folded tissue appears as a shadow and is overstained. Within the folded area, nuclei appear to be too close together.

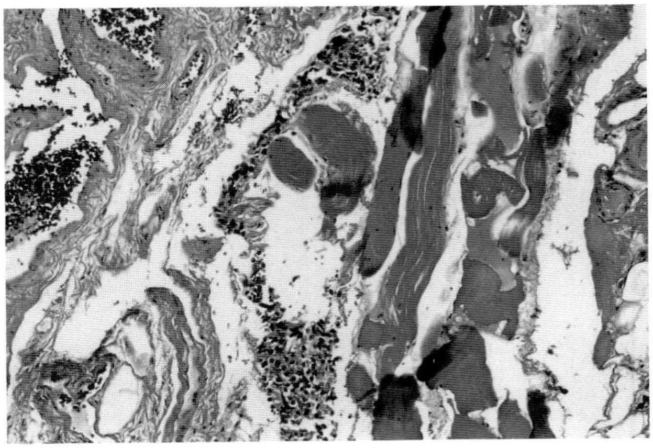

Fig. 1.28 Floater, due to knife carryover. Tumor cells are seen in tissue crevices. This section was a portion of the surgical margin in an orchiectomy performed for seminoma. The tumor was sectioned first, and some of the tumor cells from the knife filled in tissue crevices as sections of the margin were made. One can distinguish knife carryover from true marginal involvement by observing that there is no true tissue invasion by the tumor. Carryover typically only involves the edges of the tissue section.

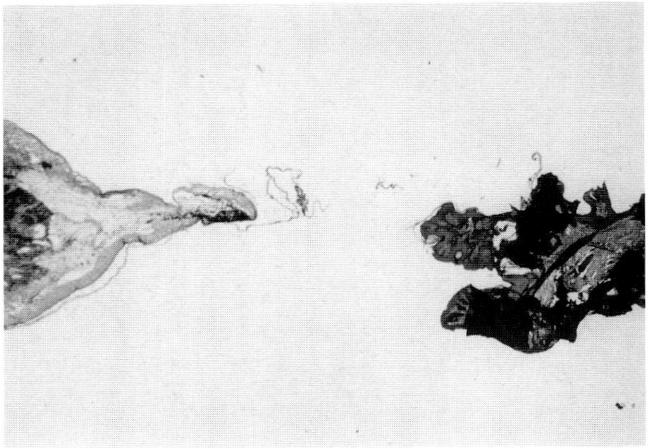

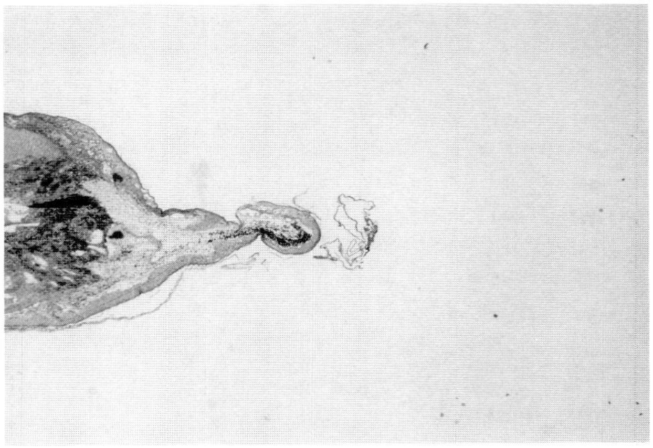

Figs. 1.29, 1.30. Floater, section of skin. This slide of a skin biopsy contains a second wrinkled fragment of skin, which is off to the side of the biopsy. The next cut of tissue (Fig. 1.30) lacks the second wrinkled skin fragment. Note that the characteristics of the two skin pieces are different. Examination of the remainder of the slides processed that day revealed a specimen, two numbers earlier, was the origin of the floater. This type of floater is usually picked up on the slide from the microtome water bath.

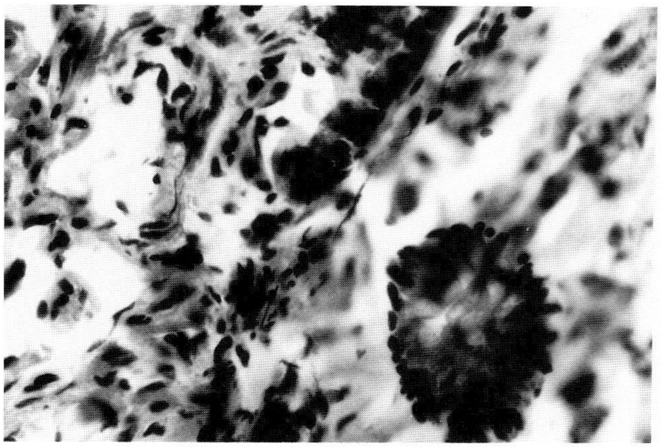

Fig. 1.31. Floater, colon. This fragment of colonic mucosa is sitting on top of a benign nerve sheath tumor. It is obviously of the wrong tissue type to be in this biopsy and can be best visualized in a different plane of focus from the underlying tissue.

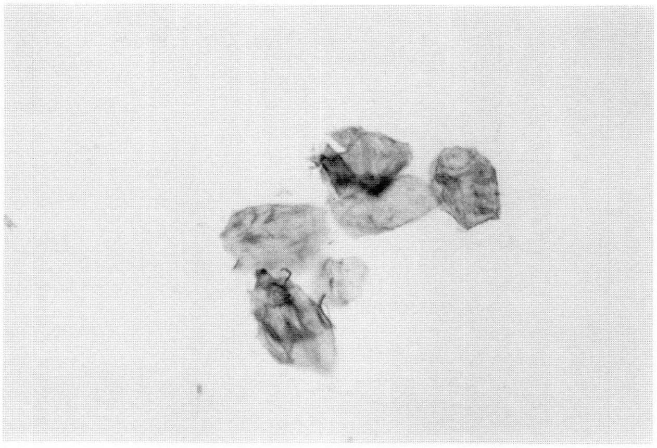

Fig. 1.32. Anucleate squames. These are typically contaminants originating from the skin of histology technicians. The squames can be anywhere on the slide and are often in a different plane of focus from the tissue sections.

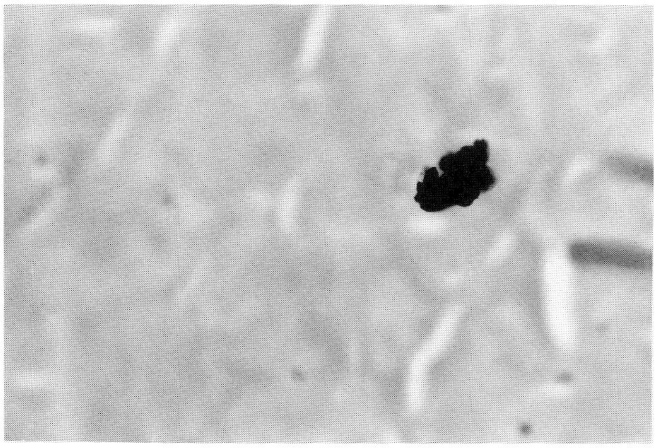

Fig. 1.33. Graphite. Graphite from pencil "lead" may be present on slides. It is usually in a different plane of focus and appears as clumps of polygonal black particles. Graphite can also truly present in subcutaneous tissue due to pencil wounds and be taken up by tissue macrophages. Graphite is weakly birefringent, particularly at its edges.

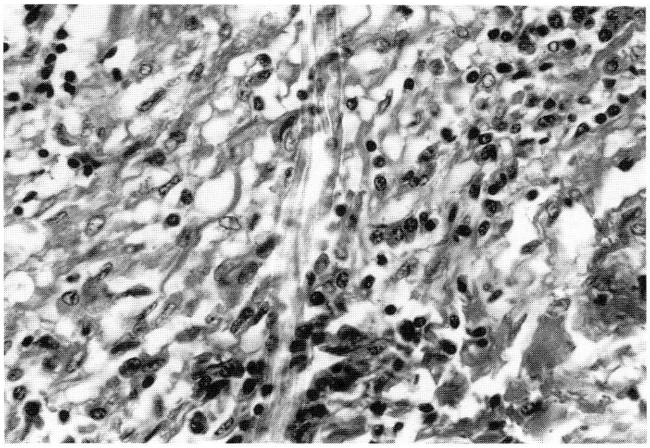

Fig. 1.34. Tissue with granulomatous inflammation and central refractile fiber. The fiber is well visualized in a different plane of focus.

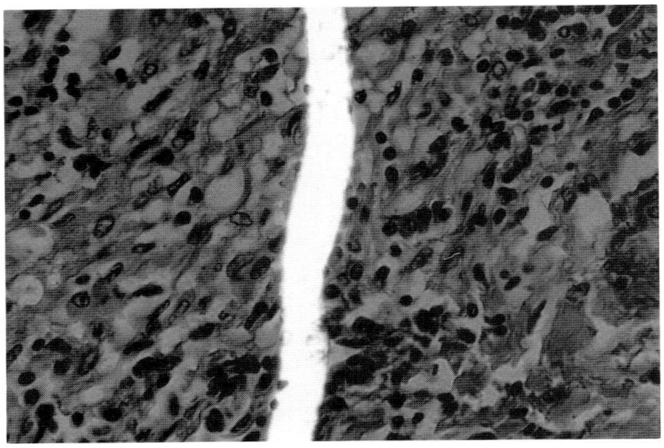

Fig. 1.35. Polarization light microscopy brings out the presence of the fiber.

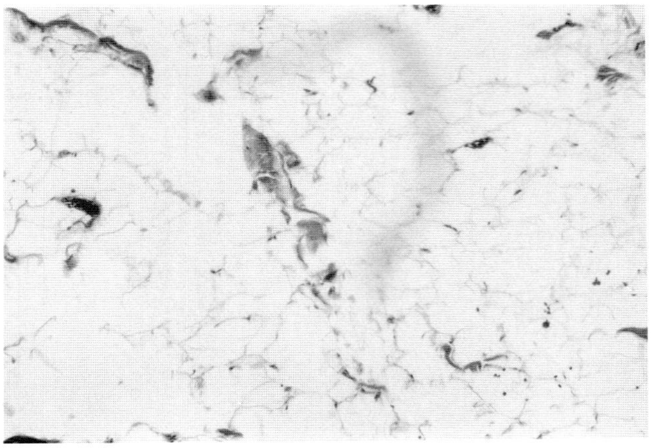

Fig. 1.36. Lint fiber, adipose tissue. The lint fiber appears as a gray shadow on routine light microscopy.

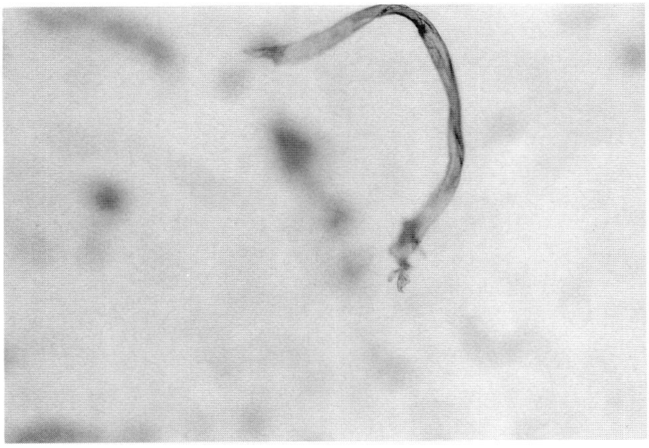

Fig. 1.37. Lint fiber, adipose tissue. The fiber comes into focus upon changing the focal plane.

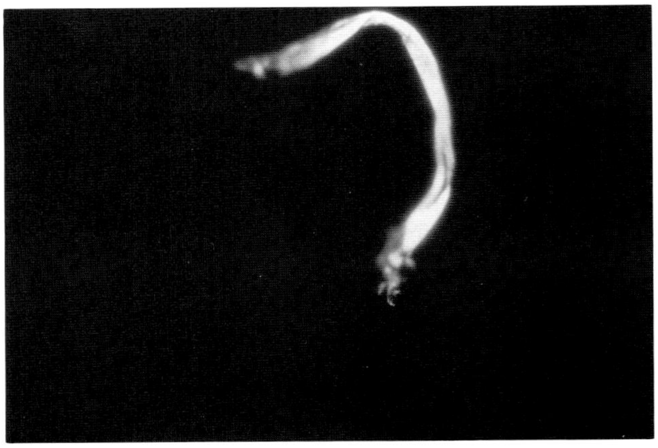

Fig. 1.38. Lint fiber, adipose tissue. The fiber is easily apparent upon polarized light microscopy.

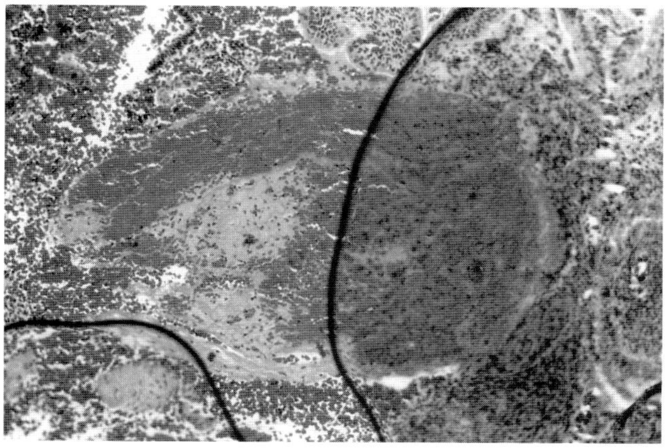

Fig. 1.39. Air bubble. Curved black lines on the slide due to air under the coverslip. Proper focusing is only possible on one side of the line.

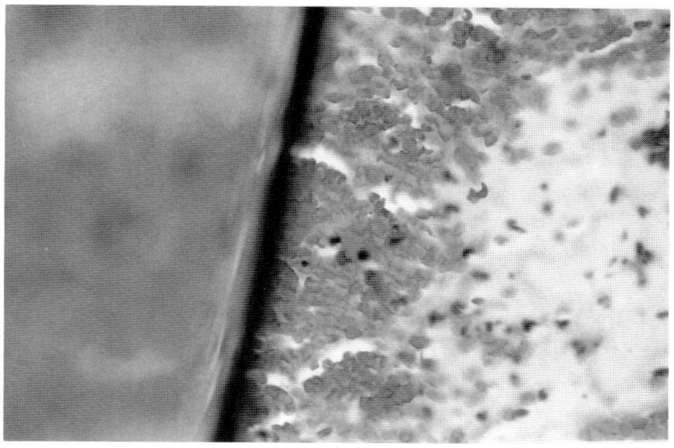

Fig. 1.40. Air bubble. High power accentuates the difference in focusing capability.

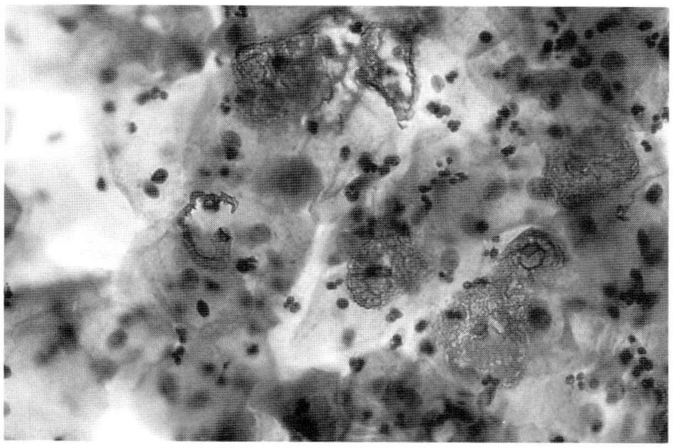

Fig. 1.41. Cornflaking, cervicovaginal smear. Air under individual cells causes dark bubbles, making the individual squamous cells appear as "cornflakes".

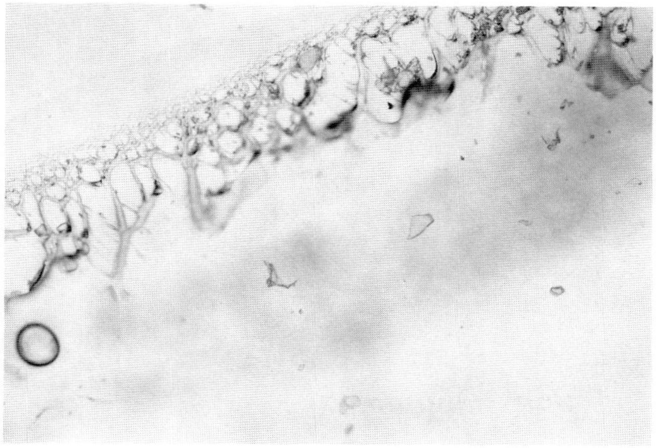

Fig. 1.42. Excess coverslip media. Edge of slide shows transparent sticky material with cracking artifact.

2

Physical and Chemical Artifacts

Tissue may undergo changes as a result of physical and chemical forces; the effects depend upon the nature of the insult. Physical changes include cellular compression (crush artifact), thermal damage, introduction of air, as well as radiation damage. Chemical changes occur with the use of drugs, particularly chemotherapeutic agents. The organs affected by drugs depend upon the mode of intake, the metabolism and clearance of the drug. The vast number of available drugs precludes a thorough discussion, and only those common agents that produce effects will be illustrated.

PHYSICAL ARTIFACTS

Crush artifact occurs when tissue is compressed either by the surgeon or the pathologist. Large specimens may show the sites of clamps by the characteristic imprint with evenly spaced parallel lines or "tooth" marks. Small biopsies frequently present as interpretation problems when the clinician uses a heavy hand in obtaining the tissue. Tissues that are most prone to showing this artifact include those without a significant supporting fibrous stroma, such as small cell carcinoma or lymphoma. Crush artifact occurs so frequently with small cell carcinoma, it is cited as a diagnostic feature. Microscopically, nuclei appear to suffer the most damage from the physical force. Nuclei are pushed together, their membranes disrupted, and basophilic material is seen streaming in different directions. Cytoplasmic membranes may be disrupted as well, with spillage of granules and other cytoplasmic contents into surrounding stroma. When marked crush artifact is present and a differential between several diagnostic entities must be made, stains for characteristic antigens or cell products may be helpful, since they are not necessarily destroyed.

Thermal injury results from a variety of sources, including iatrogenic means and accidental exposure to heat or electric current. Iatrogenic thermal injury includes usage of electrical cautery or laser beam during surgery. These types of injuries are exemplified by cervical cone biopsies, since there are several methods for obtaining a cervical cone: the "cold" knife (or traditional scalpel), the carbon dioxide laser, and the loop electric excisional conization procedure (LEEP). In recent years the LEEP procedure has gained a following among gynecologists, but not pathologists, because the interpretation of the margins is frequently compromised in a LEEP specimen. When the LEEP is performed too slowly, a relatively large thermal artifact zone is seen, rendering the entire margin uninterpretable. In addition, the traditional "cone" is compromised, with tissue frequently removed in pieces, such as the "top hat" or a variety of unintended variations. One study that measured the zones of thermal artifact produced in LEEP and laser cone procedures found the mean depth or thermal injury at ectocervical margin for the LEEP to be 0.187 mm, whereas for the laser the thermal injury zone measured 0.164 mm. This difference was more pronounced at the endocervical margin, the zone measuring 0.295 mm for the LEEP versus 0.137 mm for the carbon dioxide laser.

With accidental thermal exposures, the external examination of skin can differentiate electric from burn injury. Electrical injuries usually result in separate entry and exit current marks. Metallic particles may be detected from contact with electrical conductors, including copper, iron, zinc, and aluminum. Histologic stains for these metals will ascertain their identification.

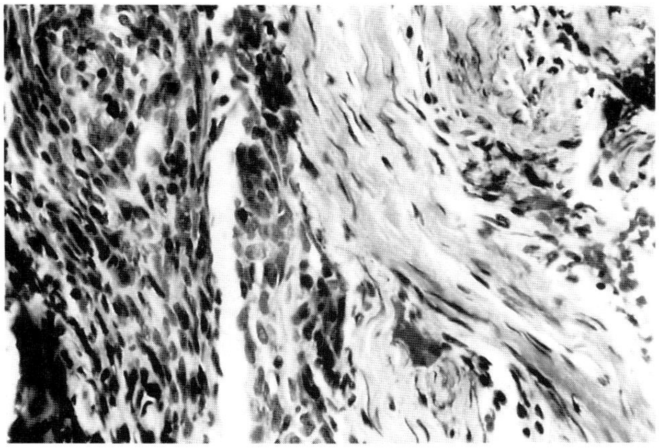

Fig. 2.1. Crush artifact, thymoma. Cells with high nuclear to cytoplasmic ratio are easily damaged by handling and exhibit crushing of nuclear material. The crushed nuclear material appears as elongated basophilic material, with nuclei pushed into each other. This artifact is most notable at the edges of the section and is particularly prominent in small biopsy specimens.

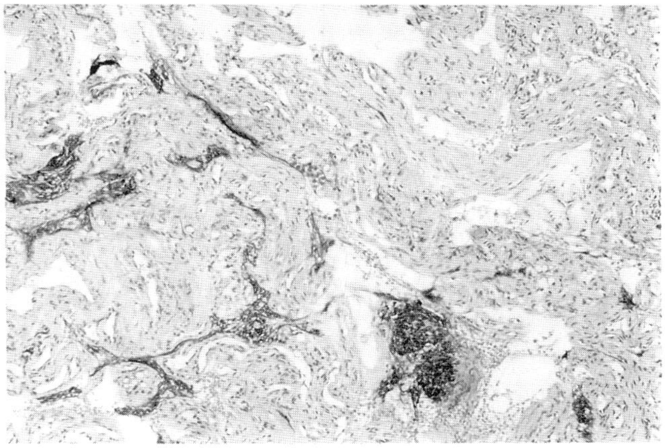

Fig. 2.2. Crush artifact, esthesioneuroblastoma. Crushed nuclear material is seen as streaks of dark material on low power, usually at tissue edges. Many tumors with small round nuclei and scant cytoplasm will show the same artifact.

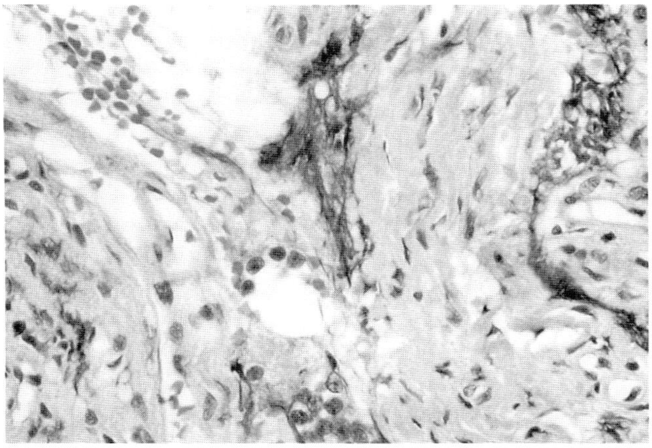

Fig. 2.3. Crush artifact, esthesioneuroblastoma, higher power.

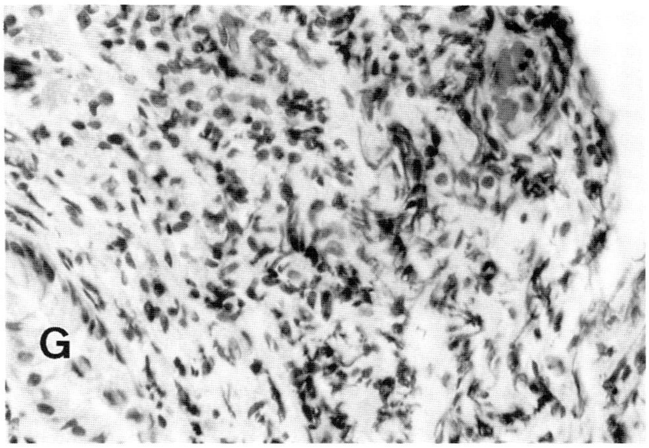

Fig. 2.4. Crush artifact, seen at edge of tissue fragment, due to forceps. Normal gland (G) and stromal tissue are seen at the opposite edge of the photograph.

Burn marks on the skin are usually in the shape of the hot object, but may be more diffuse if caused by hot flames, liquids, or gases. Histologic findings are similar. In the area suffering the most direct injury, cell necrosis occurs. In adjacent exposed areas, cytoplasm is vacuolated and nuclei are elongated. Cellular reaction includes the migration of neutrophils within 4–6 hr. Histiocytes and fibroblasts are apparent in 2–3 days, with subsequent granulation tissue formation.

Surgical suction may cause vacuoles in tissue. The negative pressure of the suction tip pulls air and mobilizes tissue fluids. Grossly, the tissue appears to be of low density and may have visible air bubbles. Blood and fibrin appear bubbly. Microscopically, this artifact appears as extracellular round spaces, whose centers may contain small amounts of fluid. In oral tissues, basophilic material, which contains acid mucopolysaccharides, has been reported in the centers, presumably pulled from myxoid tissue around dental follicles. At times, nuclei appear to line up around these spaces, and this artifact must be distinguished from true structures, such as vascular or glandular spaces. The differential diagnosis also includes soft tissue emphysema, pneumotosis intestinalis, tissue edema, gas production by bacteria, and the injection of lipids or other medications prior to biopsy. History will usually differentiate an in vivo process such as soft tissue emphysema and pneumotosis intestinalis from a surgical artifact. Prolonged periods of gas in tissues also incite a cellular reaction, including macrophages and giant cells, which will not be present in a surgically induced process. In tissue edema, individual cells are separated by fluid, without formation of air spaces. Production of gas by bacteria leads to much the same appearance as surgical suction. However, it usually occurs in tissues from infected individuals or in tissue that has been unfixed for a prolonged period prior to processing. Both Dermajet and Madajet for the injection of lidocaine cause a "Swiss-cheese" appearance of soft tissues, which usually does not distort tissue. Lipid carriers of medicinal drugs can lead to lipogranulomas. Lipid is demonstrable using Oil Red O and other special stains on tissue that has not been subjected to lipid dissolving fluids, such as xylene.

The instillation of distilled **water** into a hollow viscus prior to biopsy causes cellular edema, as occasionally happens during cystoscopy. The biopsy usually is not grossly remarkable. Microscopically, the surface epithelial cells are swollen. The depth of the cellular edema depends upon the length of time tissue is exposed to non-normal water.

The effect of **radiation** on tissue depends upon the dosage administered. Cell death occurs with high dosages, but with lesser amounts of radiation, a sequence of reactive changes occurs, which can be divided into acute, intermediate, and chronic changes. In the acute phase, there is tissue edema, endothelial proliferation, swelling of cells and collagen fibers. Ischemic effects are present due to vascular damage. In the intermediate phase, regeneration occurs. Histologically, this phase is characterized by fibrosis and the presence of pleomorphic fibroblasts. Later, during the chronic phase, the epithelium is thin and depigmented. Fibrosis is dense, and there is prominent vascularity, multinucleated giant cells, and random, pleomorphic epithelial cells. Individual cytologic changes include bi- and multinucleation, hyper- or hypochromasia, irregular nuclear contours, or macronucleoli. The cytoplasm is typically increased, but retains a normal proportion to nuclear size. Vacuolization

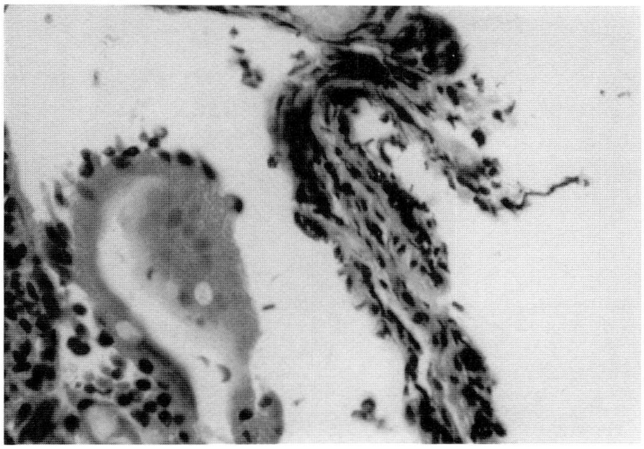

Fig. 2.5. Crush artifact, pinched tissue at the edge of duodenal biopsy, due to physical force of biopsy forceps.

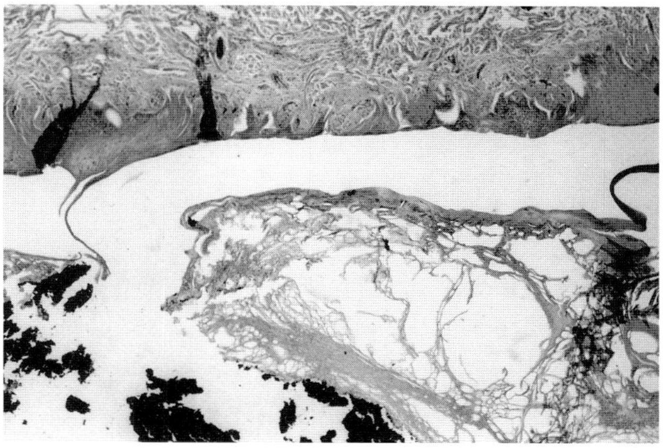

Fig. 2.6. Thermal effect on squamous epithelium. Patient suffered massive electrical burns. The tissue becomes dehydrated and is difficult to cut. Note folds in tissue.

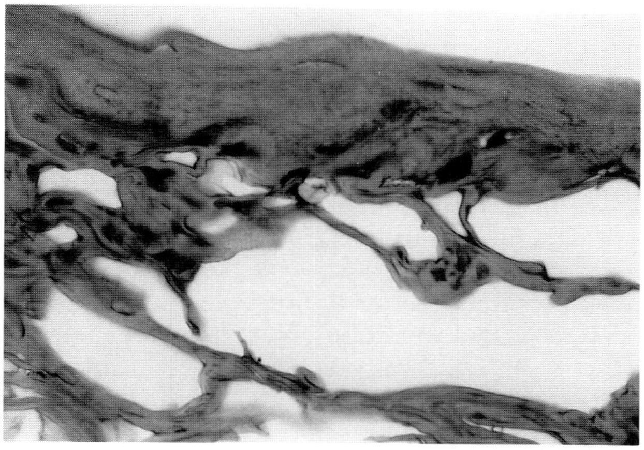

Fig. 2.7. Thermal injury. Marked tissue shrinkage and nuclear smudginess are seen in the cells.

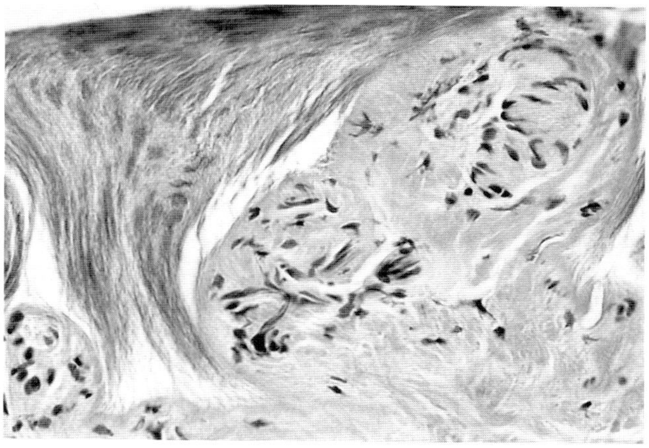

Fig. 2.8. Heat effect. The epithelium is partially separated from the underlying dermis. Increased eosinophilia of cytoplasm is seen on H&E stain. Nuclei become smudgy and elongated, sometimes perpendicular to the normal orientation.

and amphophilic staining of cytoplasm may occur, and bizarre cell shapes are not uncommon. In fact, the cellular characteristics may be so pronounced that the main differential diagnosis of radiation damage is malignancy. To differentiate, note the nuclear to cytoplasmic ratio (normal with radiation), accompanying cellular effects in adjacent granulation tissue (pronounced in radiation damage), and most importantly, history of radiation.

Other sources of energy used medically include radiofrequency current for the ablation of the atrioventricular node in the treatment of supraventricular tachycardia. Fibrosis and endocardial thrombus have been reported in a case, but no specific features of radiofrequency ablation are described.

CHEMICAL ARTIFACTS

Antineoplastic chemotherapy changes are similar to those seen in radiation. The exact chemical and its end organ determine the histologic appearance of the injury. Commonly damaged organs include lung (interstitial fibrosis, alveolar type II pneumocyte hyperplasia, hyaline membrane formation), liver (necrosis, fibrosis, cholestasis, granulomas, vascular changes), bone marrow (hypo- or hyperplasia), gastrointestinal tract (epithelial damage, ulceration), and skin (exfoliative dermatitis, allergic dermatitis, lupus-like changes). With neoadjuvant chemotherapy given for breast cancer therapy, the ductal epithelial cells undergo a random increase in size, and there is stromal fibrosis. Patient history is crucial in making the correct diagnosis.

Injectable drugs, such as insulin, heparin, and vitamin K are frequently given, but biopsies of adverse reactions are rarely obtained, since reactions are transitory and their cause obvious. Injections of insulin cause both allergic type responses, including zinc granulomas and lipoatrophy, as well as nonimmunologic responses, such as dermal scarring and hyperpigmentation. Immunizations may be associated with aluminum granulomas, in vaccines that use aluminum as a carrier, such as diphtheria, pertussis, tetanus, and influenza.

Agents may be painted on skin or mucous membranes prior to tissue excision. These agents include iodine or acetic acid solutions, which help highlight the lesion to be excised, and hemostatic agents, such as ferric subsulfate or silver nitrate.

Acetic acid is frequently used in outlining cervical or penile dysplasias or condylomata. The acid solution makes the surface of the epithelium stain more lightly than the underlying tissue.

Lugol's artifact is produced by a solution of iodine that is occasionally painted on the surface epithelium of cervices prior to biopsy to assist in the identification of areas of dysplastic squamous epithelium. Normal squamous epithelium stains brown, whereas dysplastic epithelium remains unstained. If a 5% or stronger solution is used, a microscopic artifact has been described which may hinder interpretation of the cervical biopsy. Cells become shrunken and separated from one another. There is loss of cellular and nuclear detail, with hypereosinophilia, vacuolization, and nuclear pyknosis. These findings may simulate squamous dysplasia, which can be differentiated if only well-preserved tissue is interpreted.

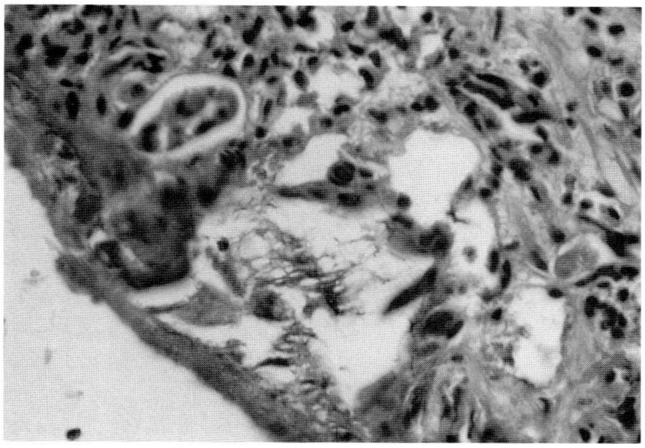

Fig. 2.9. Gastric ulcer, cauterized prior to gastrectomy (current specimen). Tissue at surface shows loss of nuclear and cytoplasmic detail.

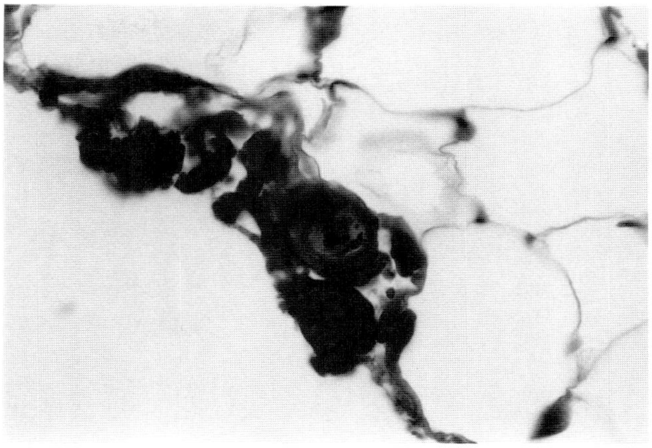

Fig. 2.10. Electrocautery effect. Fibroadipose tissue showing marked eosinophilia, condensation, and loss of cellular detail.

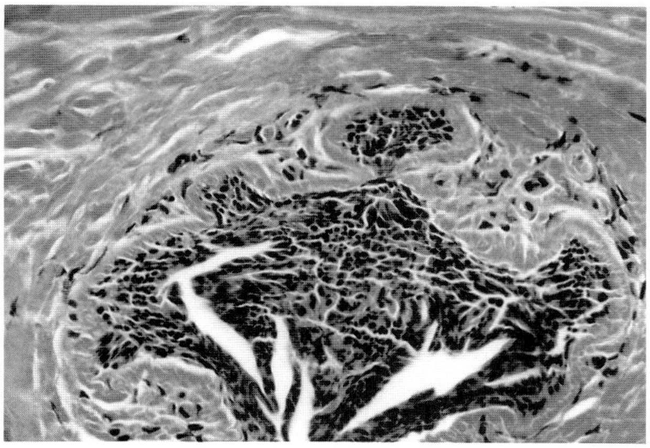

Fig. 2.11. Electrocautery effect. Duct at edge of breast biopsy, showing distortion of shape, as well as streaming of nuclei in the direction of heat effect.

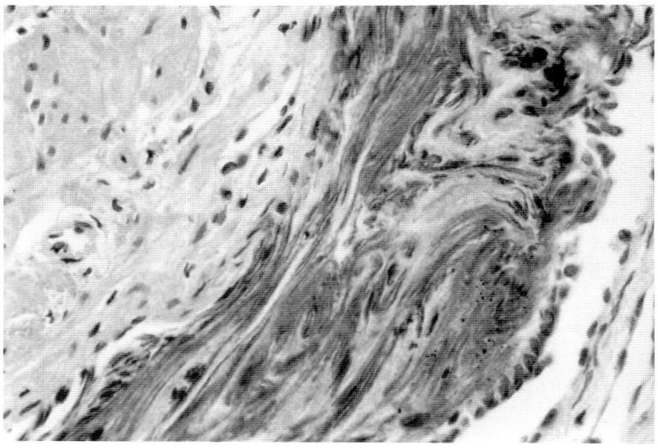

Fig. 2.12. Thermal effect at edge of section in prostate chip in transurethral resection. Stretched smudged nuclei, elongated cytoplasm.

Ferric subsulfate solution (Monsel's) is a skin and mucous membrane astringent, sometimes used for hemostasis after skin biopsy. On skin reexcisions, macrophages contain granular brown material if ferric subsulfate was used in the initial biopsy. These granules are problematic if melanoma was the primary lesion, since they mimic melanocytic granules. Reactive cytologic atypia may be present as well, further complicating the differential diagnosis. Because of its iron content, this material will be strongly positive (blue) on Perls' iron stain. Melanin will be negative for iron and positive with silver stains.

Silver deposition, after the use of silver nitrate as cauterizing agent, results in the finding of granular brown material in and between squamous ectocervical cells, sometimes in stroma in and adjacent to application areas. Like most physical or chemical damage, the exact changes depend upon the amount of exposure. In more superficial areas or glandular areas (monolayer of epithelium), the granular material tends to be in the stroma. Fibrin thrombi are frequently present in nearby vessels. The differential diagnosis of silver nitrate damage includes postinflammatory melanosis, which is the deposition of melanin pigment. Melanosis of the cervix has also been described after cryotherapy for squamous dysplasia.

Steroids are used as an anti-inflammatory agent in many sites, including intra-articular areas, soft tissues, and nasal sites. Injections of steroid material may incite localized reactions, including local allergic reactions, abscesses, secondary infections, and granulomatous inflammation. The only specific reactions are the steroid-containing granulomas, which are characterized by irregular areas of finely granular or bubbly, basophilic material (the steroid material), surrounded by histiocytes. Birefringent crystalline particles are seen by polarized light microscopy in the center of the material. The differential diagnosis on hematoxylin–eosin stained sections includes rheumatoid nodules and infectious granulomas. The demonstration of birefringent crystalline particles rules out both of these entities.

Myospherulosis refers to the finding of sac-like structures enclosing smaller endobodies, first described in nasal specimens. The clinical history typically notes hemostatic packing with petroleum-based ointment. Adjacent tissue shows fibrosis and lipogranuloma formation, with lymphocytes, histiocytes, and giant cells. Rosai has shown that the enclosed structures are red blood cells and that the outer membranes are composed of lipid. This effect can be reproduced using a lipid ointment. The limiting membrane is typically eosinophilic, as are the endobodies. The spherules are variable in size, but typically 30–100 μm, containing 5 to 7 μm endobodies. The differential diagnosis includes protothecosis, which would stain with silver, unlike myospherulosis.

Rounded bodies, known as **spironolactone bodies**, have been described microscopically in adrenal glands following spironolactone (an aldosterone antagonist) therapy. The structures are present in cytoplasm of cells of the zona glomerulosa or zona fasciculata as rounded, laminated, eosinophilic bodies, measuring 2–25 μm in size. Spironolactone bodies appear blue with Luxol blue stain. An electron microscopic study found that the inclusions are membrane-bound derivatives of the endoplasmic reticulum, not specific for spironolactone treatment, and are similar to inclusions found in other organs.

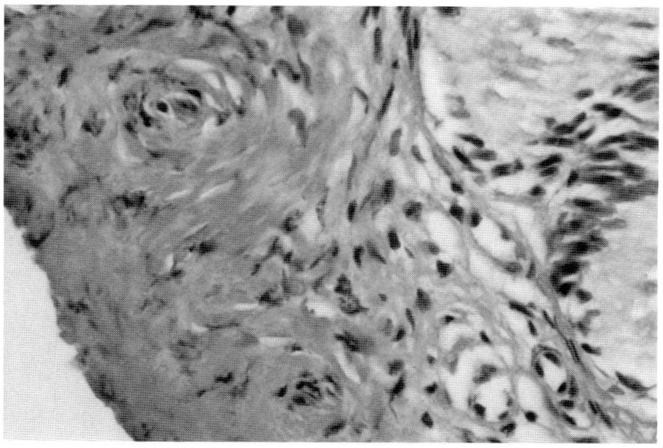

Fig. 2.13. Electrocautery effect. Cervix after LEEP cone. Tissue at edges is hypereosinophilic with separation of cells and marked nuclear distortion.

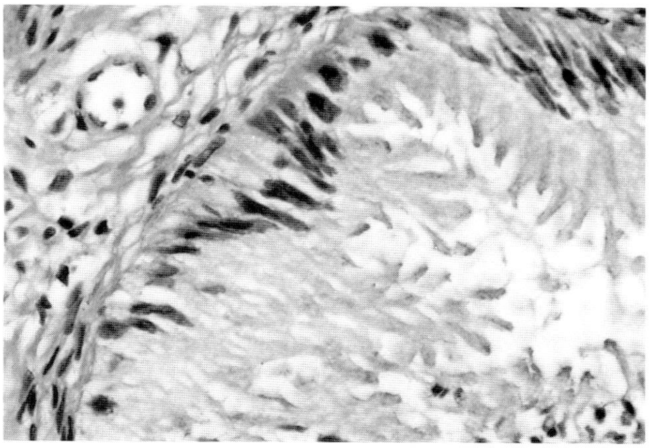

Fig. 2.14. Electrocautery effect. Cervix after LEEP cone. Endocervical glandular cells show elongation and hyperchromasia of nuclei.

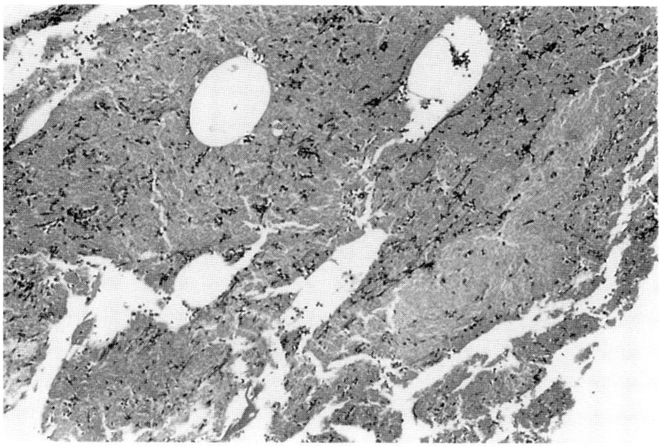

Fig. 2.15. Air suction vacuoles, brain. Soft tissue which is obtained by suction often shows oval to round air holes.

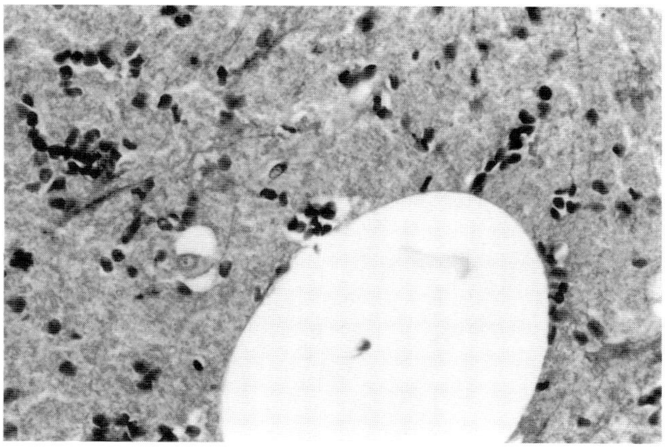

Fig. 2.16. Air suction vacuoles, brain. Note sharply demarcated hole, with no lining cells and no cellular contents.

BIBLIOGRAPHY

Baggish MS, Barash F, Noel Y, et al: Comparison of thermal injury zones in loop electrical and laser cervical excisional conization. *Am J Obstet Gynecol* 166:545–548, 1992.

Benda JA, Lamoreaux J, Johnson SR: Artifact associated with the use of strong iodine solution (Lugol's) in cone biopsies. *Am J Surg Pathol* 11:367–374, 1987.

Davenport RD: Diagnostic value of crush artifact in cytologic specimens. *Acta Cytol* 34:502–504, 1990.

Hytiroglou P, Domingo J: Development of melanosis of uterine cervix after cryotherapy for epithelial dysplasia. *Am J Clin Pathol* 93:802–805, 1990.

Lamm J, Niebyl P, Hood A: Histologic artifact due to madajet. *Arch Dermatol* 121: 835–836, 1985.

Lesack D, Wahab, Gilks CB: Radiation-induced atypia of endocervical epithelium: a histological, immunohistochemical and cytometric study. *Int J Gynecol Pathol* 15: 242–247, 1996.

Lowe DG, Levison DA, Crocker PR, et al: Silver deposition in the cervix after application of silver nitrate as a cauterising agent. *J Clin Pathol* 41:871–874, 1988.

Macaulay JC: Occupational high-pressure injection injury. *Br J Dermatol* 115:379–381, 1986.

McClatchie S, Warambo MW, Bremmer AD: Myospherulosis. A previously unreported disease? *Am J Clin Pathol* 51:699–704, 1969.

Morgan AM: Localized reactions to injected therapeutic materials, part 1, medical agents. *J Cutan Pathol* 22:193–214, 1995.

Morgan AM: Localized reactions to injected therapeutic materials, part 2, surgical agents. *J Cutan Pathol* 22:289–303, 1995.

Rosai J: The nature of myospherulosis of the upper respiratory tract. *Am J Clin Pathol* 69:475–481, 1978.

Wheeler TM, McGavran MH: Myospherulosis—further observations. *Am J Clin Pathol* 73:685–686, 1980.

Wolff M: Granulomas in nasal mucous membranes following local steroid injections. *Am J Clin Pathol* 62:775–782, 1974.

Wolfsohn AL, Green MS, Walley VM: Pathology of radiofrequency catheter ablation of the atrioventricular node. *Mod Pathol* 7:494–496, 1994.

Wysocki GP, Gusenbauer AW, Daley TD, et al: Surgical suction damage: a common tissue artifact. *Oral Surg Oral Med Oral Pathol* 63:573–575, 1987.

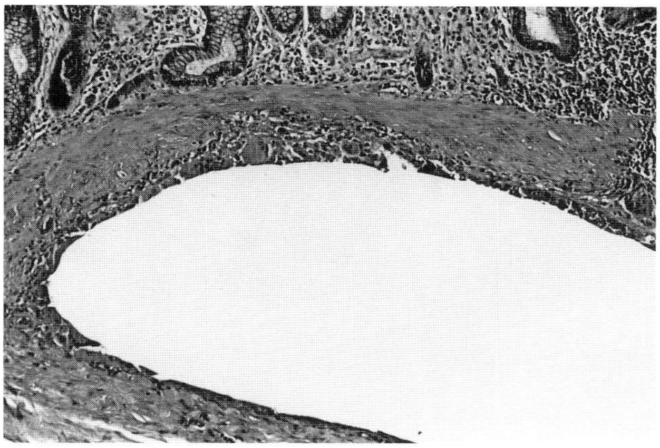

Fig. 2.17. Pneumotosis coli. Colonic epithelium and underlying oval clear space, lined by histiocytes and lymphocytes.

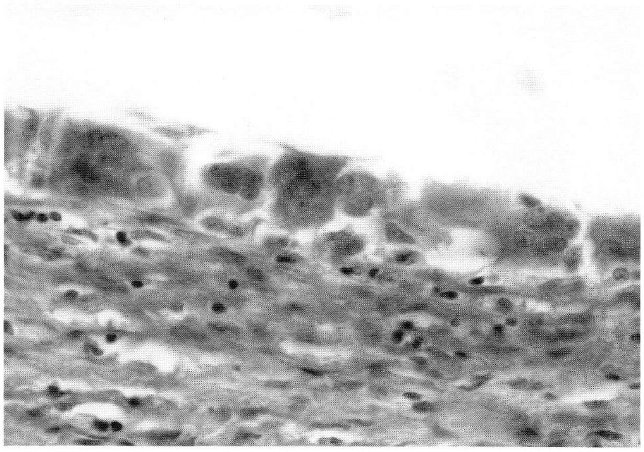

Fig. 2.18. Pneumotosis intestinalis, higher power. The vacuoles are lined by foreign body type giant cells.

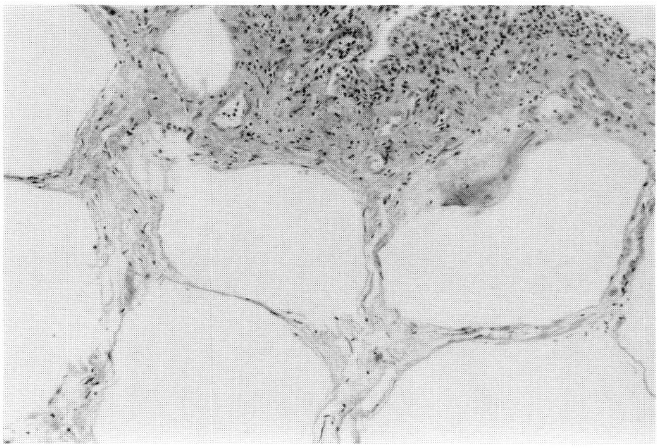

Fig. 2.19. Bladder emphysematosis. Vacuoles are simply spaces with no apparent lining cells.

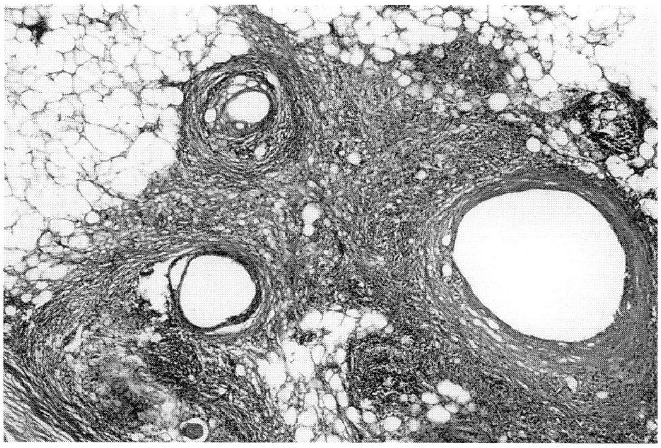

Fig. 2.20. Lipogranuloma. Large clear areas of lipid, surrounded by fibroinflammatory tissue. Note bubbly background. Lipid will be leached out on routine processing.

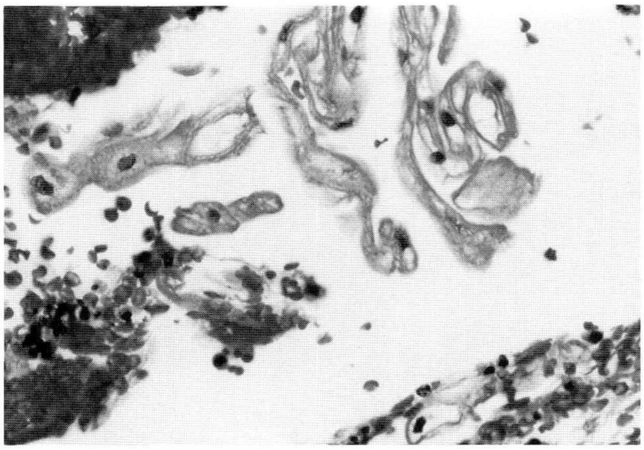

Fig. 2.21. Acute radiation damage, vagina. Ulcer debris with squamous epithelial fragments. Some of the squamous cells have hyperchromatic nuclei and perinuclear clearing, which simulates the cytopathic effect of human papilloma virus.

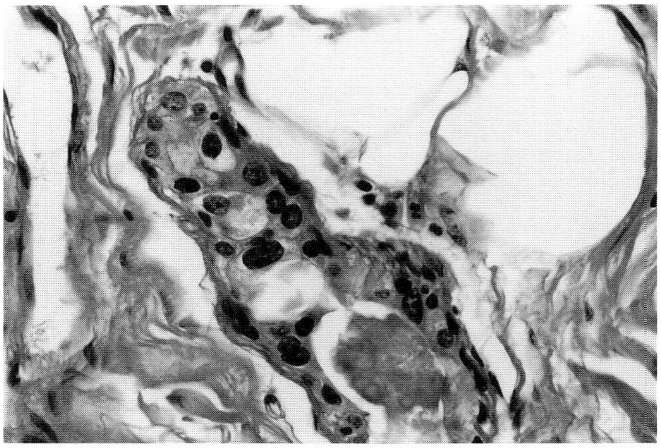

Fig. 2.22. Chronic radiation effect, breast. Ductal epithelial cells show random enlargement. Some nuclei have prominent nucleoli and others are hyperchromatic.

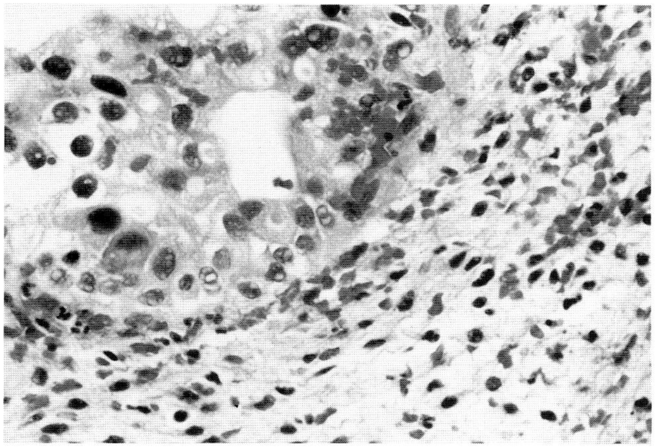

Fig. 2.23. Chronic radiation damage, bladder. The transitional epithelial cells have enlarged, hyperchromatic nuclei and vacuolated cytoplasm. Nuclear detail is difficult to discern. The underlying stroma is infiltrated by a mixture of chronic inflammatory cells.

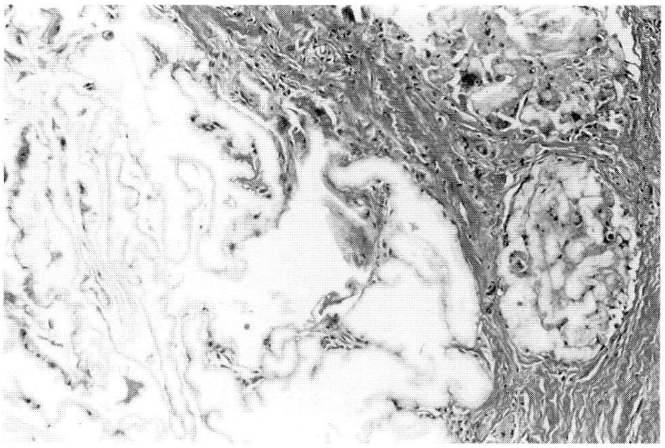

Fig. 2.24. Cystic fat necrosis in breast after radiation therapy. Fat necrosis frequently occurs in the breast after radiation therapy. The classical findings of foamy histiocytes, giant cells, and lymphocytes are not always present. After prolonged periods, areas of fat necrosis may be walled off by fibrous tissue and be centrally cystic. At times, calcified ghosts of fat cells may be apparent.

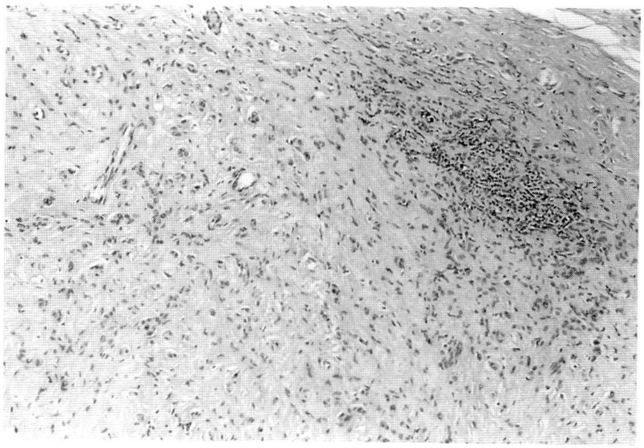

Fig. 2.25. Chemotherapy effect, metastatic breast carcinoma in lymph node. The lymph node is replaced by fibrous tissue. Only a few remaining aggregates of lymphocytes are present. Tumor cells are present as small nests.

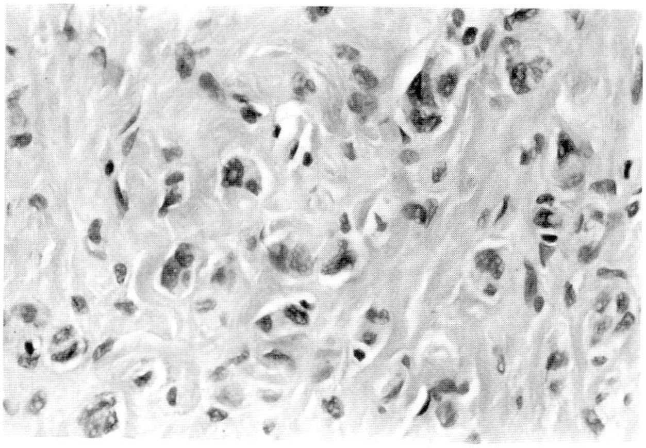

Fig. 2.26. Chemotherapy effect, metastatic breast carcinoma in lymph node. A few linear groups of tumor cells are noted. Slight separation of cells from stroma is evident. Nuclei and cytoplasm are vacuolated.

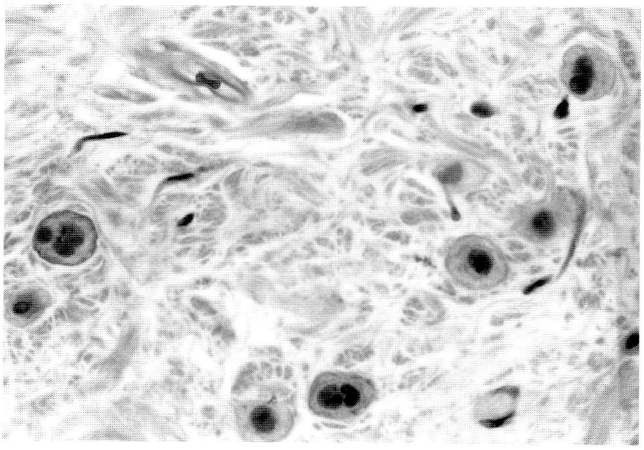

Fig. 2.27. Chemotherapy effect, breast carcinoma. Tumor cells are separated (loss of cell cohesion) and have a rounded shape. Cell membranes are prominent and cytoplasm is slightly vacuolated.

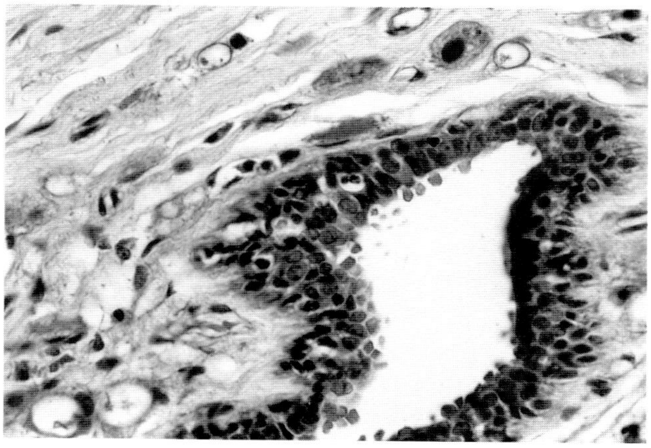

Fig. 2.28. Infiltrating lobular carcinoma of the breast after chemotherapy. Central structure is normal duct. Individual carcinoma cells outside the ducts show enlargement, cytoplasmic vacuolization, nuclear smudging, and hyperchromasia, as well as further loss of cell cohesiveness.

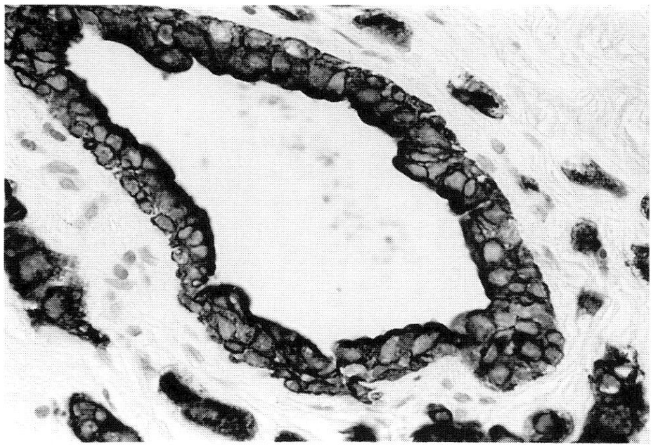

Fig. 2.29. Infiltrating lobular carcinoma of the breast, after chemotherapy. Keratin stain demonstrating retention of immunoreactivity after chemotherapy.

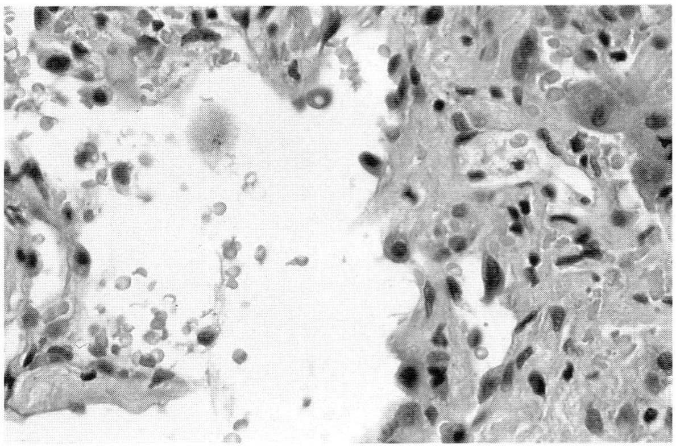

Fig. 2.30. Chemotherapy effect, lung, after bleomycin therapy. Note proliferation of Type II alveolar lining cells with cytologic atypia.

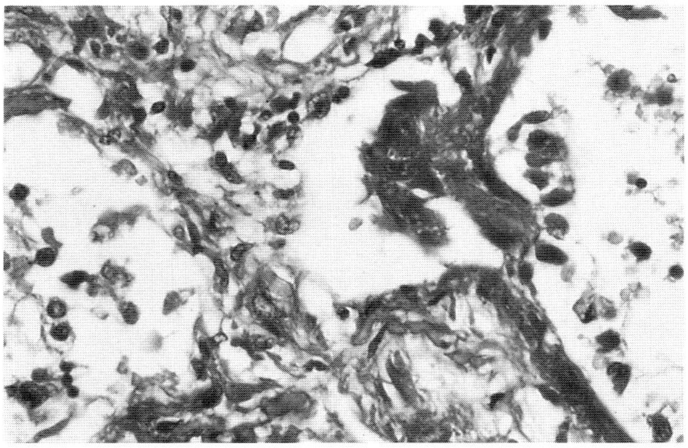

Fig. 2.31. Lung, after bleomycin therapy, Masson's trichrome stain. Fibrosis is demonstrated as blue fibers in the interstitium.

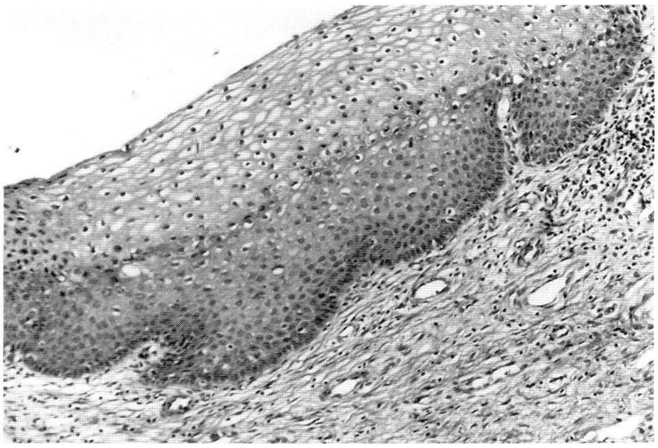

Fig. 2.32. Cervix with acetic acid effect. There is a linear artifact in the squamous epithelium, parallel to the basal layer. Cells above the line have stained lightly, with darker staining away from the surface acetic acid.

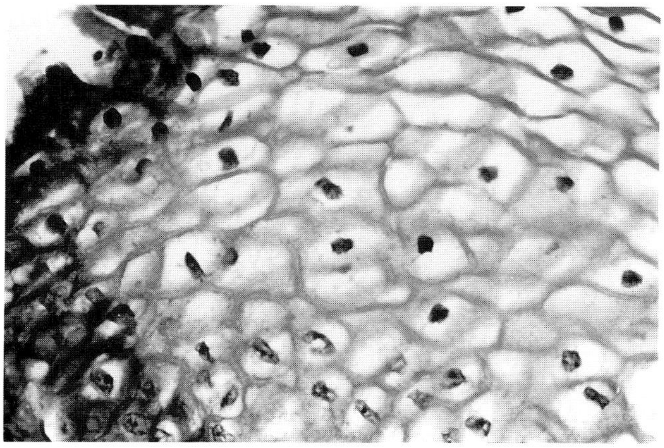

Fig. 2.33. Lugol's iodine, cervix. Dark brown-black deposits on surface squamous epithelium, with seepage around and outlining some superficial cells.

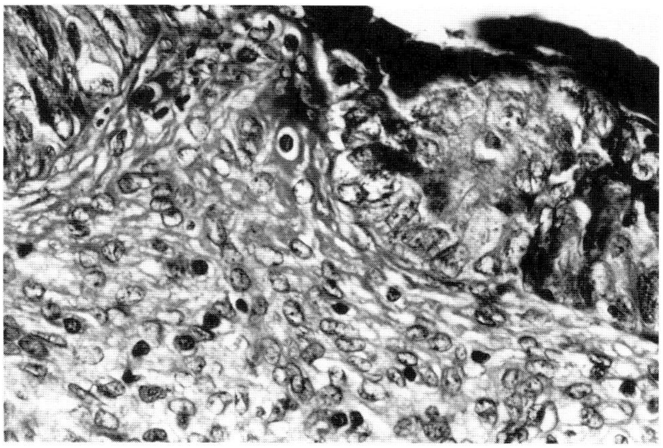

Fig. 2.34. Lugol's iodine (5%), cervix. Dark brown-black deposits on surface squamous epithelium.

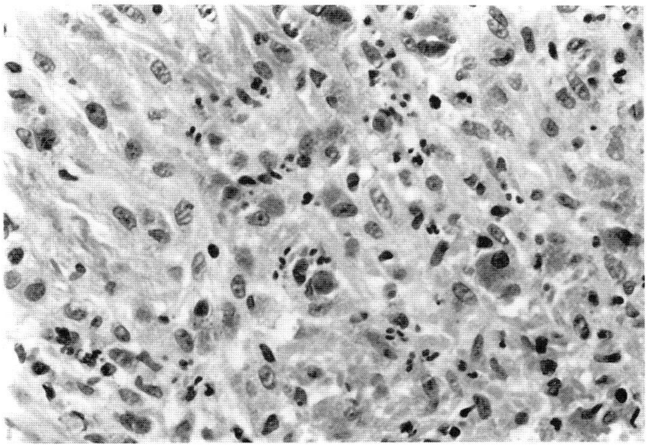

Fig. 2.35. Monsel's, solution applied to skin to stop bleeding. Note brown granules.

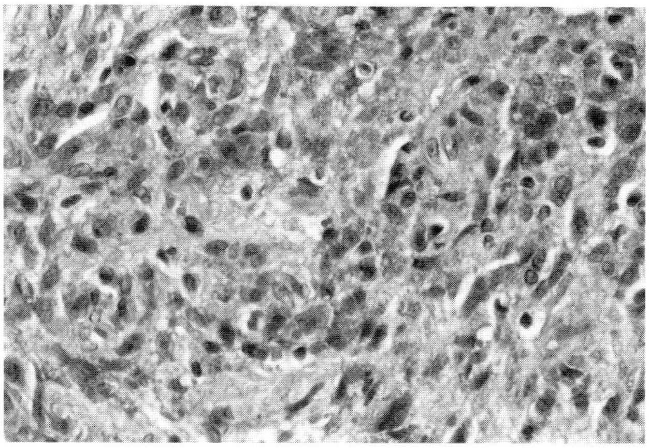

Fig. 2.36. Monsel's effect, skin biopsy site. Inflammatory fibrohistiocytic reaction, with finely granular brown material in some histiocytes.

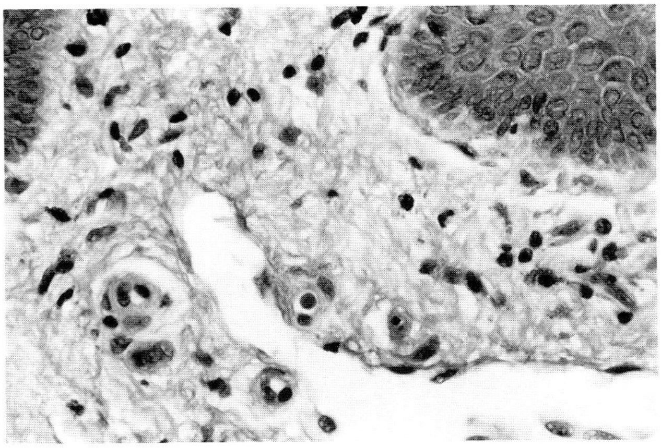

Fig. 2.37. Melanosis, skin. The dermis shows an infiltrate of chronic inflammatory cells, including melanin-containing macrophages.

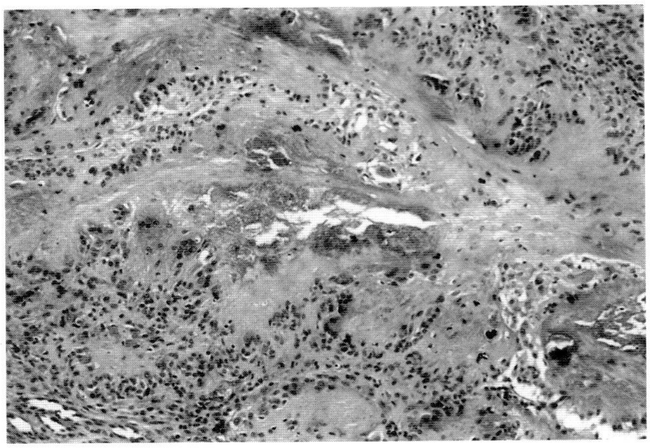

Fig. 2.38. Fibrous tissue of carpal tunnel after steroid injection. Dark granular blue-purple central matrix, surrounded by ring of histiocytes and lymphocytes.

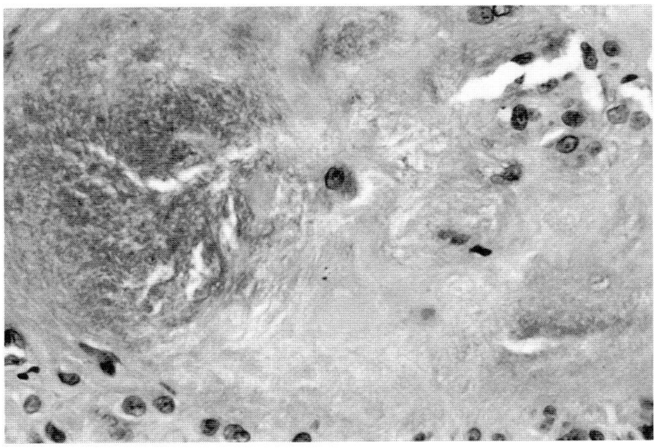

Fig. 2.39. Steroid granuloma. Note dark granular material on right, surrounded by relatively acellular matrix.

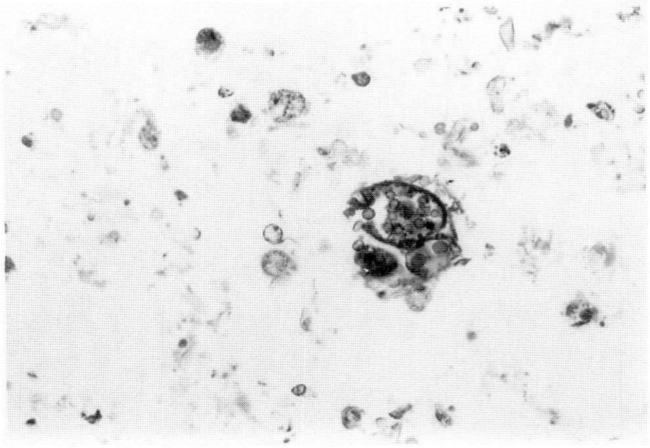

Fig. 2.40. Myospherulosis. Diagnostic area with spheroid bodies within a limiting membrane.

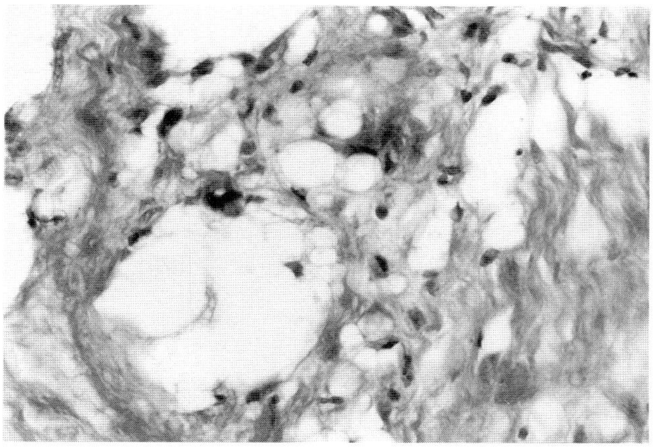

Fig. 2.41. Myospherulosis. Numerous vacuoles of varying sizes, from the injection of lipid.

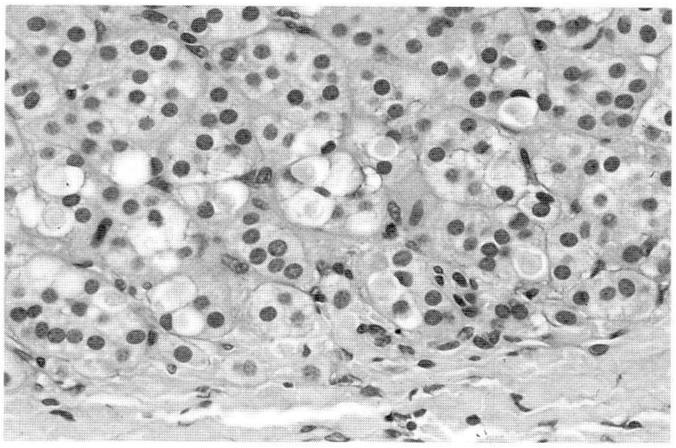

Fig. 2.42. Spironolactone bodies, adrenal. H&E stains show round intracytoplasmic bodies in the zona glomerulosa of the adrenal after spironolactone therapy.

3
Necrosis

John S. J. Brooks

Most pathologists when faced with a biopsy containing what appears to be necrotic material, quickly dispense with the case without a careful examination. Here, we describe the diagnostic significance of the various forms of necrosis and emphasize the importance of making an in-depth examination and using immunohistochemistry in certain circumstances.

Necrosis may be either a passive or an active process. In **passive necrosis,** the affected tissue is merely the recipient of a shock, a process involving a nearby tissue such as an artery. The main and perhaps exclusive example of passive necrosis is tissue infarction, usually caused by vascular insufficiency. In this form of necrosis, tissue and cellular structure is preserved. By contrast, **active necrosis** occurs as a result of a progressive tissue process which purposefully destroys cells or matrix such as collagen. Therefore, active necrosis signifies true destruction leading to tissue and cell disintegration. Examples of active necrosis include apoptosis, coagulative necrosis, and most forms of necrosis within human malignancies (although most tumors also have variable degrees of apoptosis as well).

The importance of this distinction lies in a correct and more complete interpretation of necrosis on the clinical specimen, with the result being a fuller and more clinically significant biopsy report to influence subsequent patient care.

PASSIVE NECROSIS—INFARCTION

Tissue infarction is caused by vascular occlusion phenomena and the affected tissue is thus a passive recipient of this process. Infarctive necrosis is visualized as eosinophilic material with retention of cellular and nuclear outlines. Examples include infarcted endocervical polyps, infarcted fatty tissues, infarcted chorionic villi, degenerative infarctions of uterine leiomyomas, infarction of normal lymph nodes, and infarction of nodes containing neoplasm such as lymphoma or melanoma. In practical experience, the lymph nodes so affected are frequently cervical or axillary lymph nodes, but nodes in other sites may also present an infarcted appearance.

ACTIVE NECROSIS—TYPES

Apoptosis. This is a form of active necrosis identified within tissues as individual cell necrosis. Apoptosis is constantly ongoing in most normal tissues and may be seen as karyorrhectic debris, for example, within colonic crypts or at the base of the epidermis. By this mechanism, the tissues produce a low rate of cell turnover one cell at a time resulting in replacement and renewal. The molecular biology of apoptosis involves the bcl-2 gene which regulates so-called programmed cell death. Diseases causing cell accumulation like the low-grade lymphomas have abnormalities of the bcl-2 gene. Increased apoptotic necrosis is a diagnostic feature of graft versus host disease. Apoptosis can also be identified in nearly every malignancy and is most visible in the intermediate- and high-grade lymphomas (and contributes to the "starry sky" appearance in which histiocytes contain the "tingible bodies" or nuclear fragments of degenerating cells). Examples depicted are apoptosis in colonic adenoma and in a high-grade primitive tumor. In tumors, apoptosis may be

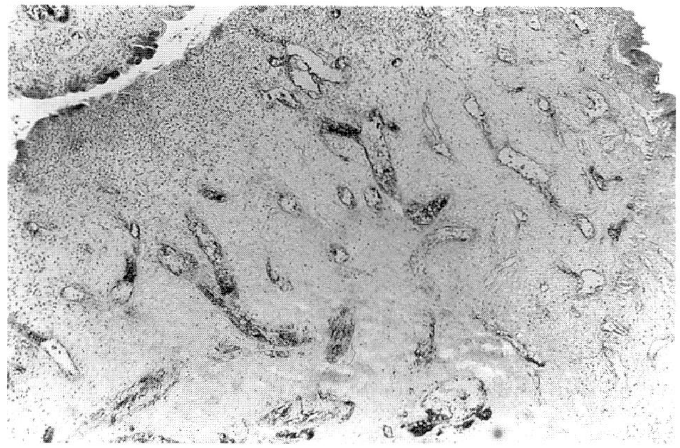

Fig. 3.1. Infarcted endocervical polyp, factor VIII immunostain. This necrotic tissue was expelled and found by the gynecologist. Examination reveals an intact vascular structure (*dark vessels decorated*), stromal tissue, rare glands, and bacterial overgrowth on the surface resembling mucin retention.

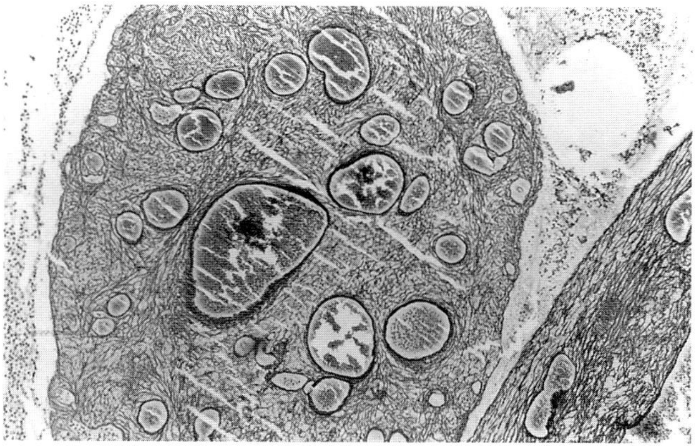

Fig. 3.2. Infarcted endocervical polyp, reticulin stain. The internal structure of the necrotic tissue is highlighted. Thus one may make a specific diagnosis of a benign polyp rather than just "necrotic" debris, which may unduly alarm the gynecologist.

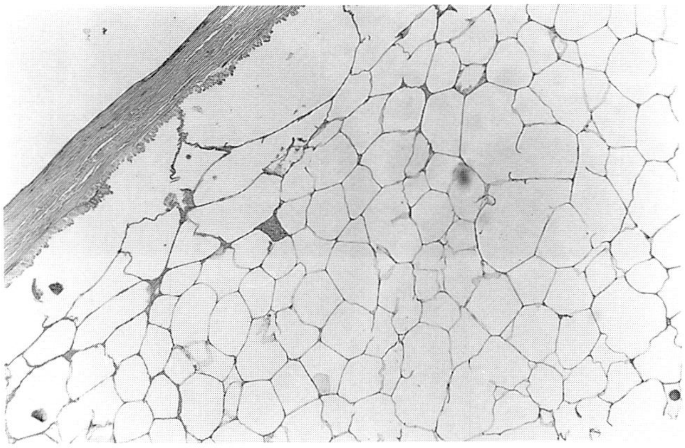

Fig. 3.3. Infarcted appendices epiploica. The adipocytes in this intra-abdominal "floater" are noted to be degenerative, at which point the cell boundaries are lost and larger lipid vacuoles are formed; such a change may occur after viability is disrupted.

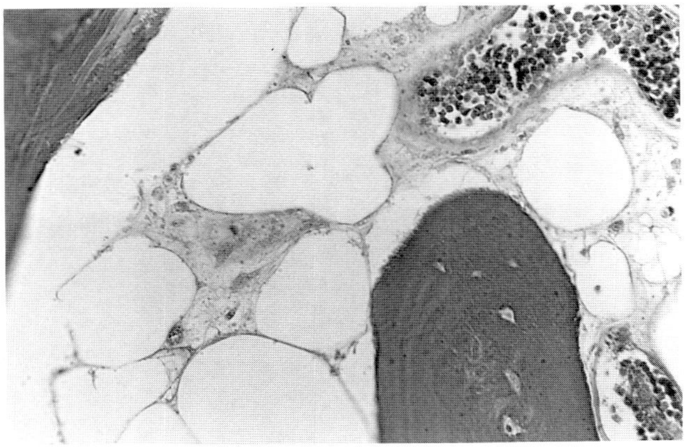

Fig. 3.4. Infarcted marrow. The fat cells lack nuclear staining, indicating necrosis; a general rule to follow is: if the fat tissue is necrotic, the bone tissue is also necrotic. This case was from an amputated diabetic foot.

inversely related to coagulative necrosis. Immunoreactivity to the bcl-2 protein has been used in the evaluation of human malignancy.

Coagulative Necrosis. This is an active process visualized as sheets of eosinophilic formless debris in tissues. At times, such debris is surrounded by palisading histiocytes (necrotizing granuloma), but it may be surrounded only by granulation tissue or foamy histiocytes and lymphocytes. At high power, the eosinophilic material can be seen to be composed of nonuniform granules and larger globules, as opposed to fibrin (see below). The most common form of coagulative necrosis is the "necrotizing" granuloma of tuberculosis. Other infectious diseases exhibit this feature as is well known. However, of more interest here is the coagulative necrosis noted in human malignancies, and again there is no form to the eosinophilic debris.

Combined Active/Passive Necrosis. In human malignancies, a combination of types of necrosis is often seen: apoptosis to a variable degree, coagulative necrosis in many lesions, and occasionally infarctive-type passive necrosis. This explains why, in areas of active necrosis, some areas retaining intact cellular borders like infarction may be noted; such areas are useful in determining the cellular composition of the necrotic debris.

DIAGNOSTIC EVALUATION OF NECROSIS

Frequently necrotic material is received in pathology, either in the form of a needle biopsy or a more generous biopsy specimen. Such material can be expelled per vagina or coughed up, the result of an endobronchial tumor being disrupted. Certainly, a diagnosis of "necrotic debris" is helpful and points the clinician to the necessity for retrieving additional tissue for proper diagnosis. However, there are situations in which proper evaluation of the necrotic material may render a highly suggestive diagnosis.

Attention to the internal detail of the necrotic material may reveal features as mentioned above. First, one is encouraged to carefully examine the hematoxylin–eosin section for areas in which cellular form may be preserved. Secondly, at high power, examine the cell size and shape, as well as the size of nuclei and presence of nucleoli. Next, architectural features should be reviewed. If as a result of this examination, a neoplasm is suspected, immunohistochemical stains should be performed (see below).

Evaluation of pure coagulation necrosis is not always possible. Sometimes, as in necrotic lung due to an infection, the architecture on a reticulin stain is still visible, but the content and nature of the cellular infiltrate is lost. Only areas of infarctive necrosis contain the necessary intact cell form to be evaluated by techniques such as special stains (reticulin stain) and immunohistochemical stains. Thus, in tumors, one needs to search for areas within the coagulated debris for the possibility of infarcted areas combined with it. It is important to recognize that antigens are still preserved in many examples of infarcted tissue and infarcted tumors.

When the necrotic tissue fails to disclose any identifiable structures or cellular debris, one should order recut slides in the hope of identifying either viable areas or evaluable necrotic material with somewhat preserved cellular structure.

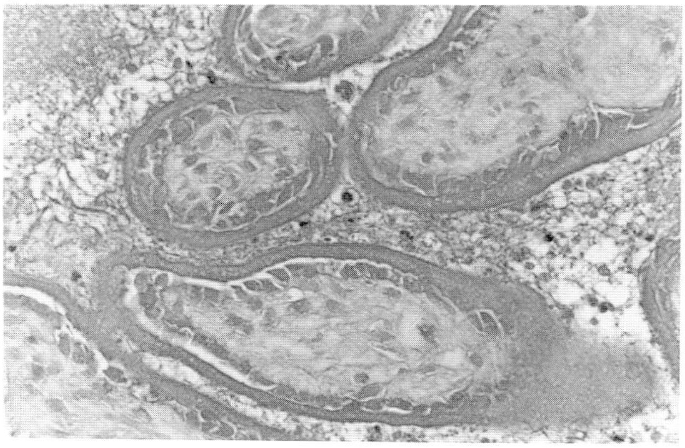

Fig. 3.5. Necrotic chorionic villi. These infarcted villi are nonetheless visible, with complete retention of structure; this finding in endometrial curettings excludes the presence of an ectopic pregnancy. The trophoblastic cells will react with cytokeratin and human chorionic gonadotropin (HCG).

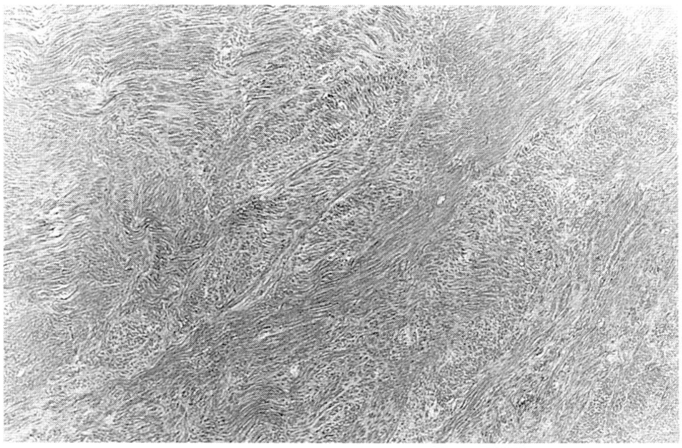

Fig. 3.6. Infarcted neoplasm, leiomyoma. In this uterine myomectomy specimen, the cells show retention of form indicative of an infarctive type of necrosis.

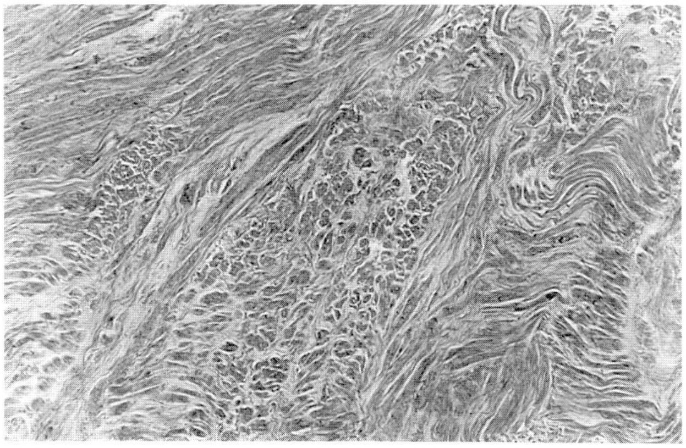

Fig. 3.7. Infarcted neoplasm, leiomyoma, high power. The alternating fascicular pattern is visible, as are extremely pale elongated nuclei. Cells themselves are not disrupted nor are nuclear fragments present, as would be the case in coagulative necrosis.

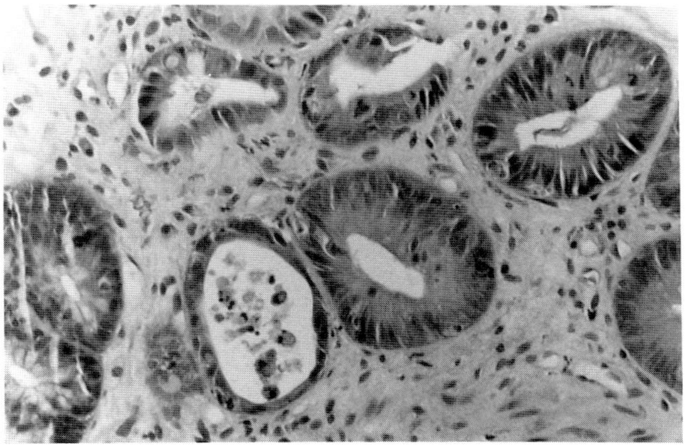

Fig. 3.8. Graft versus host disease (GVH), colonic biopsy. Nuclear karyorrhectic debris is noted both within dilated, damaged crypts (*center*), and at the basement membrane as aggregated material (*upper right*).

When lymph nodes become infarcted or involved with necrotic tumor, the result is often a mass surrounded by a dense fibrous rim. The histologic response to necrosis within a lymph node may take the form of nonpalisading clear foamy histiocytes and scattered lymphocytes within the fibrous walled reaction. Careful attention to the infarcted material may reveal either normal structures or abnormal features such as nests of tumor cells. Frequently, the overall size of the infarcted nuclei can be appreciated, including whether or not nucleoli are present. Importantly, a reticulin stain will still be reactive within the necrotic tissue, highlighting any pattern such as normal architectural features including vasculature or the presence of tumor nests.

The quantity of necrosis can be important to assess in addition to the cellular content. Estimation of the percent of necrosis is useful diagnostically in the evaluation of certain tumors. For example, a high (>90%) necrosis has a predictive value in terms of survival in the patient with osteosarcoma. In some instances, particularly when evaluating specimens after chemotherapy has been given, necrotic tumor debris may be seen. In such cases, it is important to make a diagnosis of "no viable tumor seen" even though the necrotic outlines of tumor may be visible; this statement adds more information than just declaring "necrotic debris in lymph nodes". Such might be the case with germ cell tumors, lymphomas, or osteosarcoma subjected to chemotherapy prior to removal, and a properly worded report reinforces the intended effectiveness of the therapy to the clinician.

Use of Immunohistochemistry on Necrotic Lymph Nodes. When one is faced with a necrotic lymph node, whether infarctive or coagulative type, one may utilize standard markers such as leukocyte common antigen (LCA), L26 (CD20), UCHL1, and other markers to delineate the pattern of staining. Such reactions will allow visualization of normal but obscured structures such as germinal centers, mantle zone cells, and T zones. By comparison with normal nodal architecture, one may obtain a sense of whether the lymph node is normal or abnormal. This approach would be analogous to the ability to obtain gene rearrangement data on necrotic nodes.

Aside from lymphoid markers, many other antibodies will decorate necrotic cells, including epithelial markers like cytokeratin, endocrine markers like chromogranin, and mesenchymal markers like vimentin and desmin. It is worthwhile to attempt such staining to delineate the potential malignancy even when no viable areas are identified. A word of caution is in order: areas of complete cellular disintegration may give a background stain with some, but not all markers; these tend to be markers that are also present in serum or blood like factor VIII related antigen or α_1 antichymotrypsin. One should evaluate regions on the slide with some degree of intact cell form.

To give some idea of the clinical usefulness of immunohistochemistry on necrotic tissue, the following instance is related (but not depicted): a mediastinal mass was resected and noted to be composed of a completely necrotic nodule. In a number of areas, cellular outlines were visible and two cell sizes could be discerned. This case was diagnosed as a necrotic thymoma with the assistance of immunohistochemistry. Sheets of epithelial cells were identified using cytokeratin, and the smaller cells proved to be lymphocytes which retained their staining with LCA and were also demonstrated to be of T-cell origin using UCHL-1, as should be the case with a thymoma as opposed to a

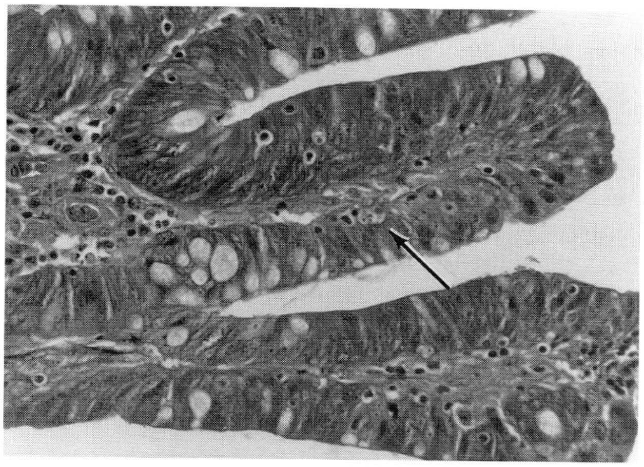

Fig. 3.9. Apoptosis in tubular adenoma of colon. Small clusters of nuclear karyorrhectic debris (*arrow*) are noted in one portion of this tubular adenoma, along with larger round nuclei identifiable as lymphocytes.

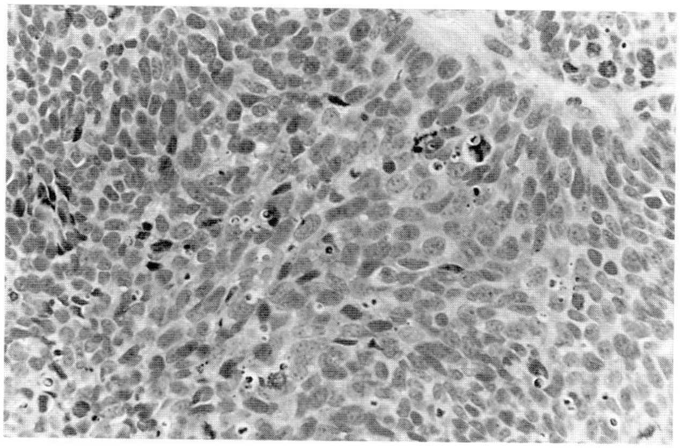

Fig. 3.10. Apoptosis in small round cell tumor. Highly mitotic tumors such as lymphomas and primitive neuroectodermal tumors (PNET, here) often contain karyorrhectic debris indicating apoptosis.

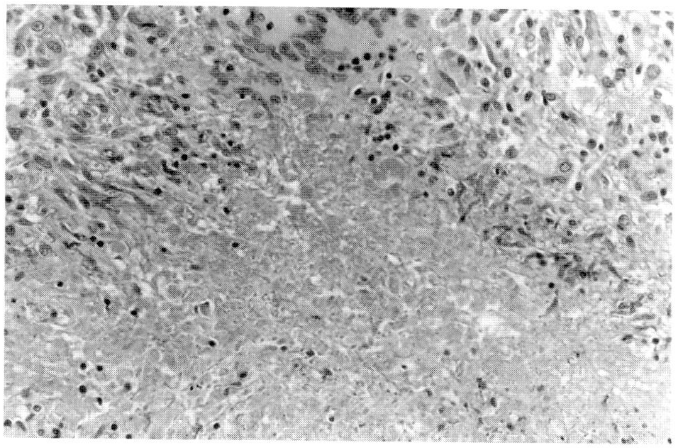

Fig. 3.11. Necrotizing granuloma. The necrotic debris (*bottom*) is surrounded by palisading histiocytes and a Langerhans' giant cell. Note the presence of variably sized granules and dark nuclear fragments from karyorrhexis.

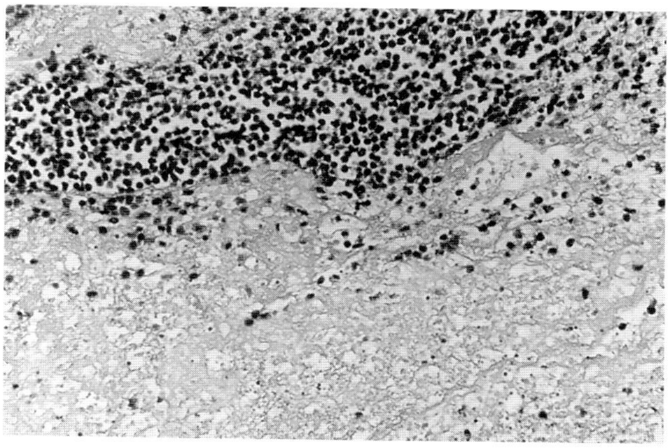

Fig. 3.12. Mixed or combined necrosis: infarcted lymph node. Several weeks after a prior surgery, this material was found floating free in the abdominal cavity. Its nature can be determined to be a lymph node containing necrotic small lymphocytes (*top*) and coagulative debris (*bottom*). Only the former intact cells will contain interpretable immunoreactivity.

metastasis to a lymph node. Thus, the clinicians were given a specific diagnosis and the patient could be assured that the completely resected tumor was a noninvasive type requiring no further therapy.

DIFFERENTIAL DIAGNOSIS OF NECROSIS

Fibrin. Because of its eosinophilic staining pattern, fibrin can be mistaken for necrotic material. This is particularly possible when a hematoma is encountered or in bronchial biopsies where aggregates of fibrin can mimic necrotic tumor cells. However, at high power, fibrin can be distinguished from necrotic debris by attention to detail: fibrin has a fine fibrillar structure and lacks the grain-like or globular nature of true tumor necrosis. It almost always has a uniform appearance in contrast to the variability of granules in necrotic cellular material.

Mistaking fibrin for necrotic debris is probably the most common error and can lead to an unnecessary workup for malignancy.

Fibrin can be confirmed with the histochemical stain phosphotungstic acid–hematoxylin (PTAH) or by an immunohistochemical stain using antifibrin or fibrinogen.

Fibrillar substances. As a fibrillar substance, collagen also stains with eosin and, under the proper conditions such as a fragmented biopsy, may be mistaken for necrotic debris. A trichrome stain will separate the two substances as collagen will be bluish and fibrin unstained (red).

Amyloid. In a fine needle aspiration or fragmented biopsy, amyloid can be mistaken for necrosis. Again, attention to the firmer nature of amyloid and lack of variable granularity will aid in the differentiation. When in doubt, a histochemical stain for it such as Congo red can be performed.

Cooked Foreign Material. Rarely, one will encounter pieces of cooked food in a pathology specimen. We have seen fragments of meat in the bronchus which, due to the cooking process, appeared as eosinophilic coagulated material. The internal structure of muscle could be discerned after closer inspection.

BIBLIOGRAPHY

Aihara M, Truong LD, Dunn JK, et al: Frequency of apoptotic bodies positively correlates with Gleason grade in prostate cancer. *Hum Pathol* 25:797–801, 1994.

Arends MJ, McGregor AH, Wyllie AH: Apoptosis is inversely related to necrosis and determines net growth in tumors bearing constitutively expressed *myc, ras,* and HPV oncogenes. *Am J Pathol* 144:1045–1057, 1994.

Buja LM, Eigenbrodt ML, Eigenbrodt EH: Apoptosis and necrosis: basic types and mechanisms of cell death. *Arch Pathol Lab Med* 117:1208–1214, 1993.

Castle VP, Heidelberger KP, Bromberg J, et al: Expression of the apoptosis-suppressing protein *bcl*-2, in neuroblastoma is associated with unfavorable histology and N-*myc* amplification. *Am J Pathol* 143:1543–1550, 1993.

Colgan TJ, Pendergast S, LeBlanc M: The histopathology of uterine leiomyomas following treatment with gonadotropin-releasing hormone analogues. *Hum Pathol* 24: 1073–1077, 1993.

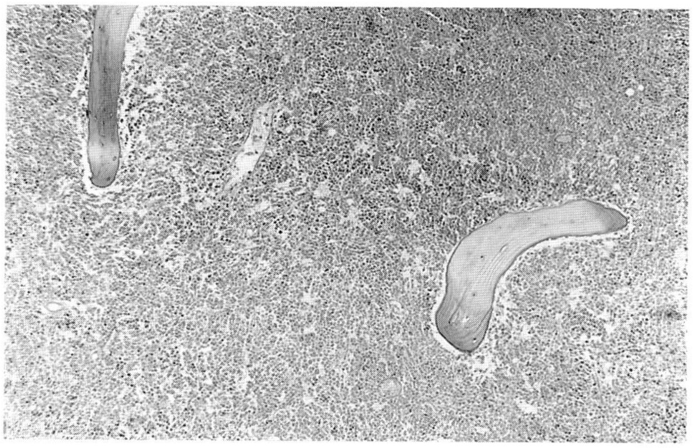

Fig. 3.13. Necrotic leukemia in marrow. A fairly specific diagnosis can be made on this highly cellular bone marrow showing complete necrosis without fat.

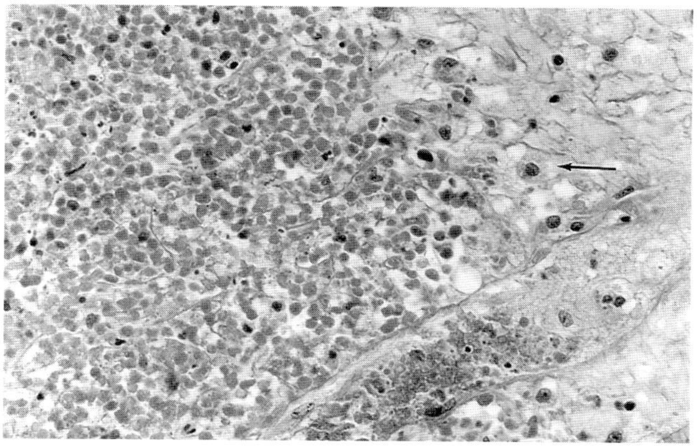

Fig. 3.14. Necrotic leukemia in marrow, high power. The necrotic cells are noted to have uniform nuclei (unlike chronic myelocytic leukemia [CML]) and nucleoli; the nuclei approximate the size of nearby histiocytes (*arrow*), thus consistent with blastic cells of acute leukemia, lymphoblastic in this case.

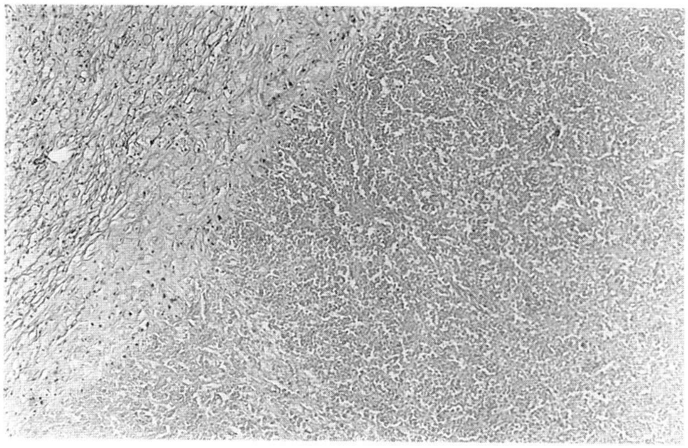

Fig. 3.15. Necrotic lymphoma. This completely necrotic (infarcted) lymph node lacks normal architecture and appears replaced by a neoplastic proliferation. No structures like germinal centers are seen.

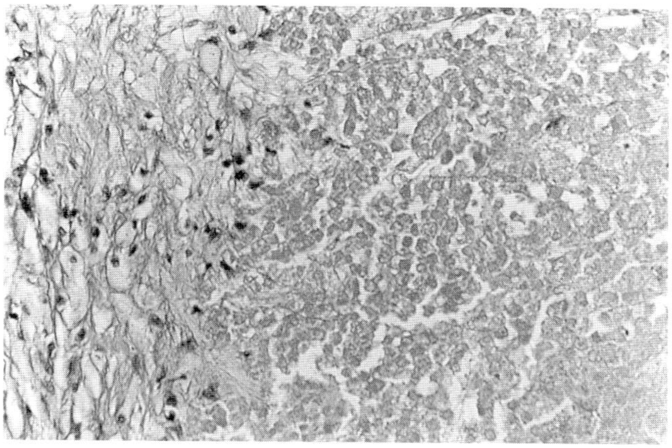

Fig. 3.16. Necrotic lymphoma, higher power. By comparison with small lymphocytes, the necrotic cells are larger and grow in sheets suspicious for lymphoma. Note that the nuclear structure of the cells is visible and nucleoli are present.

Farber E: Programmed cell death: necrosis versus apoptosis. [Review]. *Mod Pathol* 7:605–609, 1994.

Kerr JFR, Winterford CM, Harmon BV: Apoptosis: its significance in cancer and cancer therapy. *Cancer* 73:2013–2026, 1994.

Laszewski MJ, Belding PJ, Feddersen RM, et al: Clonal immunoglobulin gene rearrangement in the infarcted lymph node syndrome. *Am J Clin Pathol* 96:116–120, 1991.

Misdorp W, Hart G, Delemarre JFM, et al: An analysis of spontaneous and chemotherapy-associated changes in skeletal osteosarcomas. *J Pathol* 156:119–128, 1988.

Norton AJ, Ramsay AD, Isaacson PG: Antigen preservation in infarcted lymphoid tissue. A novel approach to the infarcted lymph node using monoclonal antibodies effective in routinely processed tissues. *Am J Surg Pathol* 12:759–767, 1988.

Oren M: The involvement of oncogenes and tumor suppressor genes in the control of apoptosis. *Cancer Metastasis Rev* 11:141–148, 1992.

Pezzella F, Gatter K: What is the value of bcl-2 protein detection for histopathologists? *Histopathol* 26:89–93, 1995.

Schimke RT, Mihich E: Fifth annual Pezcoller Symposium: apoptosis. *Cancer Res* 54:302–305, 1994.

Shapiro SH, Sohn LC: Rapid microwave phosphotungstic acid–hematoxylin stain for paraffin and glycol methacrylate sections. *J Histotechnol* 17:125–126, 1994.

Staunton MJ, Gaffney EF: Tumor type is a determinant of susceptibility to apoptosis. *Am J Clin Pathol* 103:300–307, 1995.

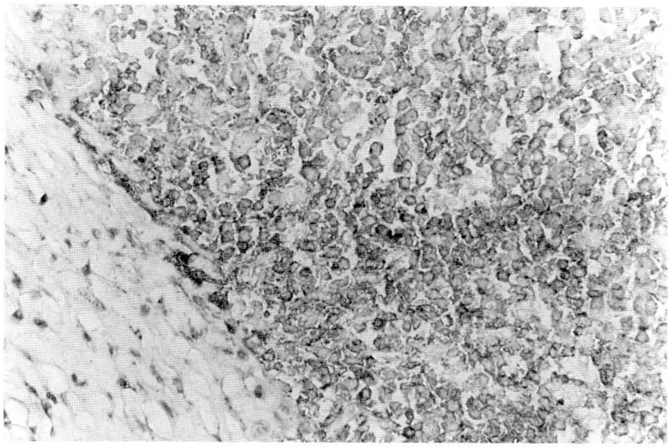

Fig. 3.17. Necrotic lymphoma, leukocyte common antigen immunostain. Immunoreactivity is noted in this large cell lymphoma with positive membrane staining around large nuclei. This tumor also typed as a B-cell neoplasm.

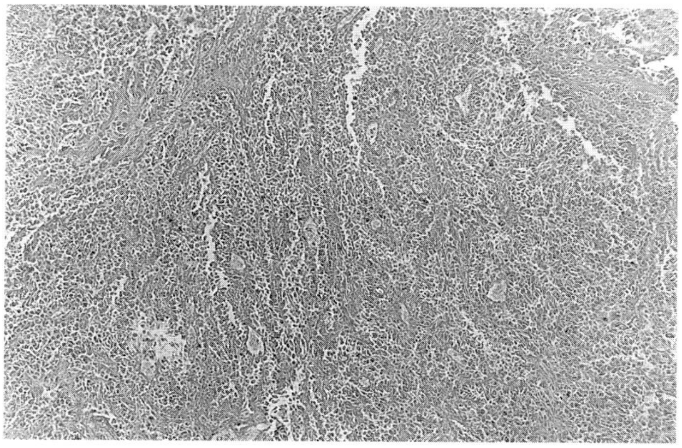

Fig. 3.18. Necrotic carcinoma in axillary lymph node. This node contains necrotic tissue suggestive of tumor. Note the presence of elongated nests of tumor and blood vessels.

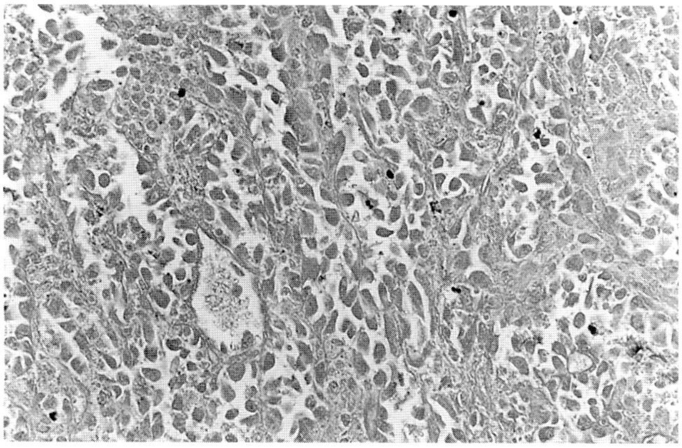

Fig. 3.19. Necrotic carcinoma in axillary lymph node, high power. The nuclei are larger than those of endothelial cells.

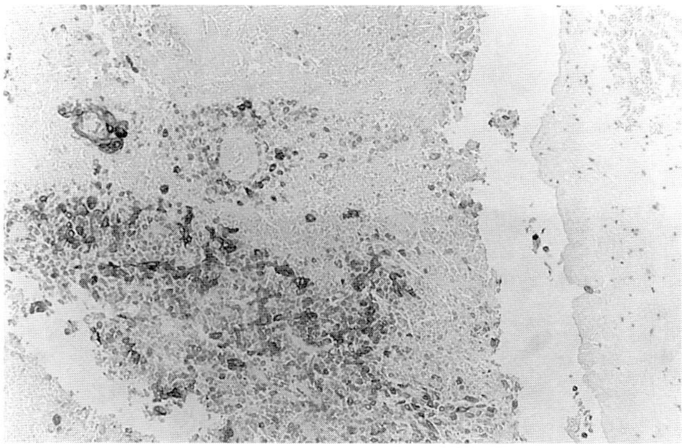

Fig. 3.20. Metastatic carcinoma, axillary lymph node, cytokeratin stain. With the lymph node capsule at the right, note many cytokeratin-positive tumor cells.

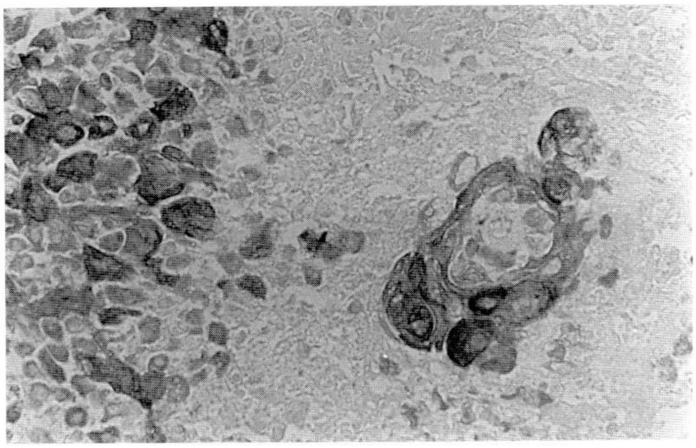

Fig. 3.21. Metastatic carcinoma, axillary lymph node, cytokeratin stain, high power. Cytokeratin reactivity highlights the growth pattern and delineates the amount of cytoplasm present. Even pearl formation can be detected (*right*). Further history determined that this patient had squamous cell carcinoma of the lung.

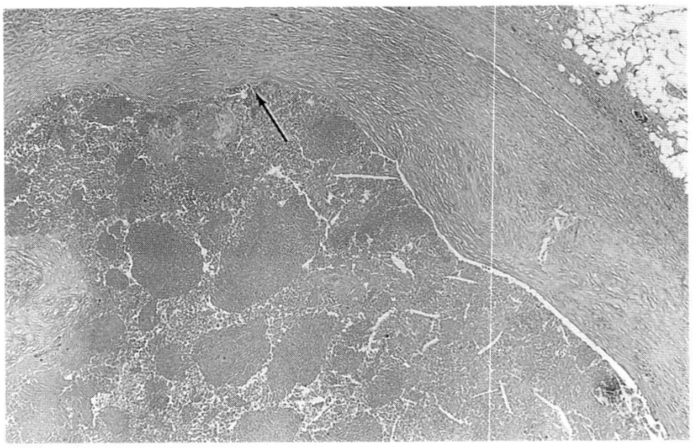

Fig. 3.22. Necrotic axillary mass. In the original slides, this material appeared to be totally necrotic; however, recuts disclosed focal viable tumor (*upper center, arrow*).

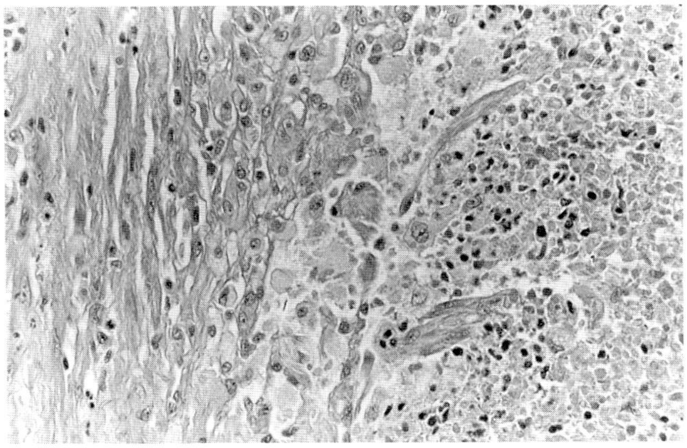

Fig. 3.23. Frequently, necrotic deposits are surrounded by a rim of foamy histiocytes and a fibrous reaction; this can be seen in nodes bearing necrotic lymphoma and metastatic melanoma, and can also occur around a necrotic normal node.

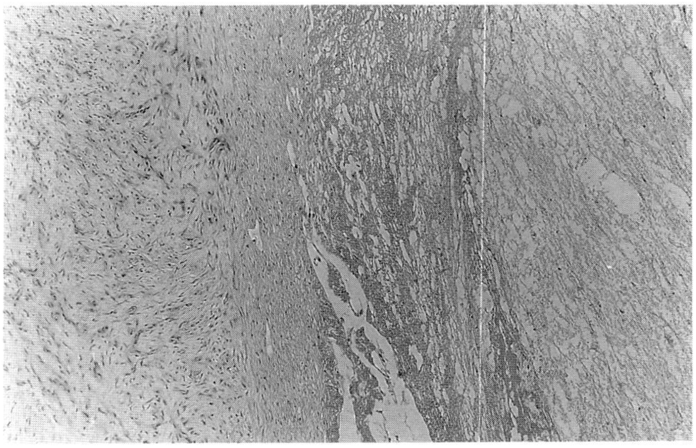

Fig. 3.24. Fibrin. At medium power, fibrin (*left*) can be associated with granulation tissue (*right*) from the site of prior surgery.

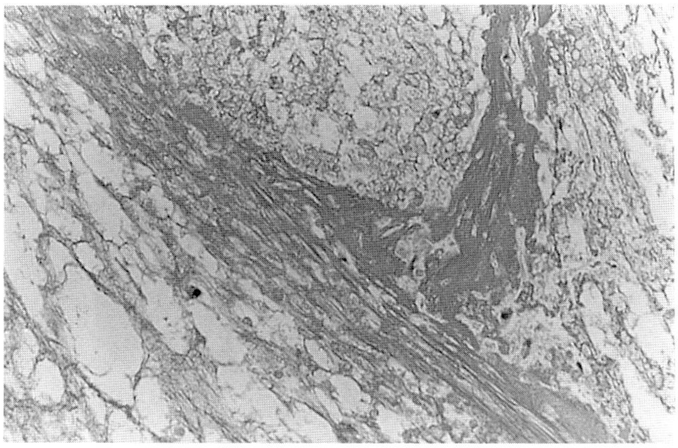

Fig. 3.25. Fibrin, high power. Fibrin can mimic necrotic debris but has a fine uniform granularity when dense (*center*) and a fibrillar matrix when loose (*periphery*).

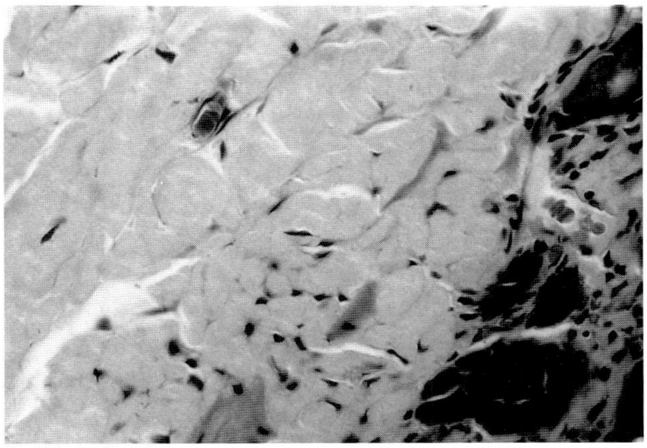

Fig. 3.26. Amyloid, small bowel. Note thick wavy collections of hyaline fibers. The fibers are uniform, without granularity.

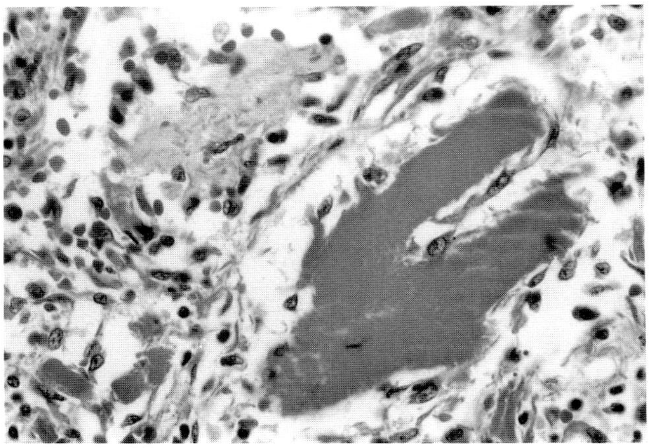

Fig. 3.27 Cooked meat. The meat appears as densely eosinophilic, slightly granular material with peripheral nuclei. Ghost outlines of internal nuclei are not present. This material is typically found in the gastrointestinal tract or the lungs, due to aspiration.

4

Medical Biomaterials

Biomaterials include processed, naturally occurring biologic substances, synthetic polymers (plastics), dyes, minerals, and metals. This chapter will discuss naturally occurring biologic substances and synthetic polymers based on their primary medical application. Dyes are discussed in the pigmented materials chapter, and most of the minerals and metals are discussed in a separate chapter. Because of the wide variety of currently available medical biomaterials and the constant additions of new materials, this chapter can only touch upon some of the more common biomaterials that may be encountered.

Naturally occurring biologic substances may be derived from either plant or animal sources. Some commonly encountered substances include cellulose, collagen, fibrin, and silk. Products containing cellulose, silk, and collagen will be birefringent. However, many animal products are not easily identified by special techniques, since they are similar to human tissues.

Synthetic polymers include fluorocarbons, silicones, polyurethane, and polyamides/polyethylenes/polypropylenes. To identify synthetic polymers, polarized light microscopy is helpful, because these substances have oriented molecular structures and thus are birefringent. Most plastics appear orange to red with Sudan stain, especially after prolonged exposure to stain (24–48 hr). Specific identification may use differences in solubility, as there is relatively little differential staining with available methods. The fine structure of plastics can be seen on scanning electron microscopy.

In time, biomaterials may either be absorbed or show signs of mechanical wear. Absorption of materials is through the usual biologic processes, including phagocytosis, proteolysis, or hydrolysis. The effect of mechanical wear is associated with changes in the physical characteristics of the material, such as material loss, fragmentation, or hardening. With fragmentation, biomaterials may provoke a foreign body reaction, serve as an infective nidus, or even embolize in the case of vascular prostheses.

Pathologic calcification in biomaterials is a major cause of failure of the material and limits their use. Examples of biomaterials that are affected by pathologic calcification include bioprosthetic heart valves, mechanical blood pumps, intrauterine contraceptive devices, and contact lenses. Calcification may occur within material, adjacent tissue, or blood elements and tends to occur along flexing surfaces. In fact, emboli formed after vascular prosthesis are usually caused by calcific debris, not larger tissue fragments.

VASCULAR GRAFTS, TISSUE REINFORCERS, AND RECONSTRUCTIVE MATERIALS

There has been a diversity of materials used in the surgical reconstruction of vessels, beginning with Vinyon-N cloth in the early 1950s. **Dacron**, a trademark name for a special **polyester** material, was introduced in the 1970s and is now used almost exclusively in vascular grafts. Grafts constructed of Dacron may be either knitted or woven. Woven grafts are not usually incorporated into surrounding tissues, and their luminal coverage is incomplete. With time, blood flow may be inhibited by thrombus formation due to the irregularity in collagen coverage within the lumen. Incomplete incorporation also leaves foci prone to bacterial infection.

Knitted Dacron double velour grafts have the advantage of more uniform adherence to surrounding tissues, due to more complete incorporation by

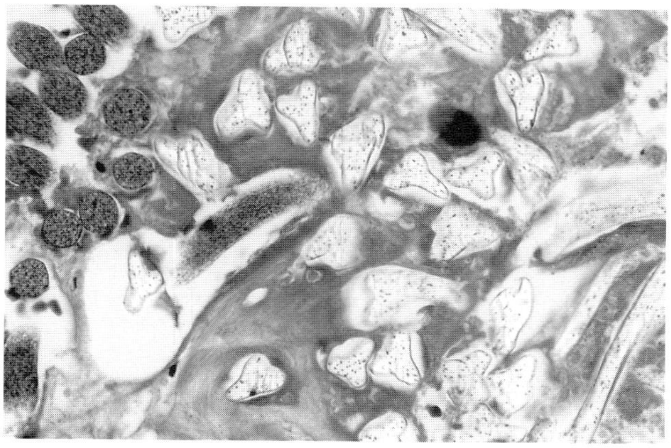

Fig. 4.1. Woven Dacron graft, after 10 yr. Cross-sectional view of round and triangular fibers, as well as a partial longitudinal view.

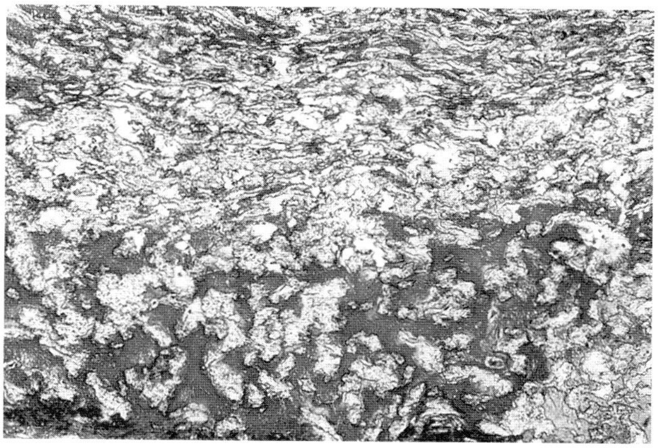

Fig. 4.2. Gortex graft material. Irregular refractile clear material, in wavy aggregates.

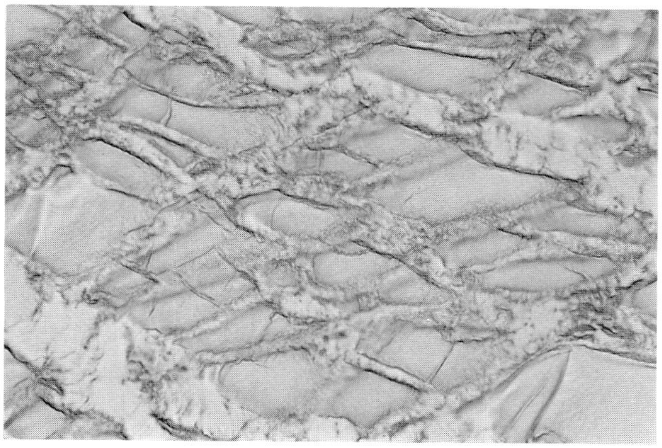

Fig. 4.3. Gortex graft. Refractile clear polygonal shapes, laid down in tile-like pattern.

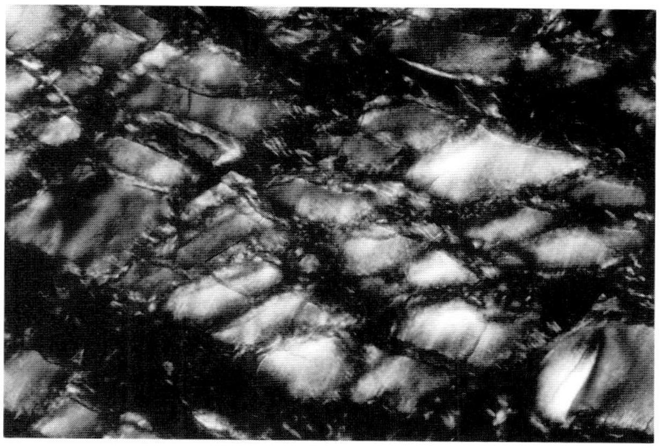

Fig. 4.4. Gortex graft, polarized light.

fibroblasts. These grafts are typically used in the abdominal aorta, as well as in the reinforcement of the gastrointestinal tract, abdominal wall, etc. Microscopically, Dacron graft material is composed of numerous uniform, round filaments. Small, relatively uniform black granules are present within the filaments. Colored fibers are used to mark positions for the surgeon and have a higher density of black granules. The material is refractile and is easily polarizable. The tissue reaction to Dacron double velour grafts is characterized by an initial phase in which the graft is embedded in a layer of fibrin. An organizational phase occurs during the ensuing weeks to months, in which a dense fibrous capsule is formed on the graft exterior, as well as a proliferation of fibrous tissue within interstices of the graft. A mixed chronic inflammatory response accompanies the fibrous proliferation, including histiocytes, foreign body giant cells, lymphocytes, plasma cells, and eosinophils. Capillaries also proliferate. At the anastomotic site, fibrosis forms slightly earlier and is denser than in the remainder of the graft. The final phase is seen after a year, in which the graft is fully incorporated in fibrous tissue with a mild chronic inflammatory response. Atherosclerotic plaques may form in graft lumens after prolonged time intervals.

Polytetrafluoroethylene (PTFE, Teflon, Gortex) is an extremely high-molecular-weight substance and one of the most inert of biomaterials. It is employed for a variety of surgical usages, such as arterial lines, prosthetic bypass grafts, tissue reinforcers, catheter sheaths, and pledgets. PTFE has different appearances, depending upon the form.

When used in woven grafts, PTFE adheres poorly to surrounding tissues. Anastomotic aneurysm formation has been described with Teflon grafts; if ruptured, dissection and/or death may ensue.

Reinforced PTFE (Gortex) appears as a rubber-like sheet of opaque material that is typically used as a tissue reinforcer. Microscopically, Gortex is composed of irregular clear fragments with minute uniform anisotropic granules. The material may appear as interconnecting fine strands.

A paste form of PTFE, Polytef (polytetrafluoroethylene, glycerin, and polysorbate mixture), is used in paralyzed vocal cords to increase turgor. The Teflon may migrate to draining lymph nodes and has been reported to migrate distally to the lungs as well. The acute cellular reaction to Teflon includes infiltration by polymorphonuclear leukocytes (PMNs) with abscess formation. A chronic histiocytic, granulomatous response with fibrous capsule formation ensues with more prolonged exposure. Grossly, Polytef appears as a yellow pasty material. Microscopically, Teflon is a slightly yellow, clear refractile material with rod-like or fractured crystal-like (flake) shapes. These fragments are variably sized, and may be seen as clumps up to 100 μm or more. On polarized light microscopy, Teflon is highly birefringent and may give off a slight blue color. Definitive identification of the material may be made by infrared absorption spectrophotometry on tissue sediment after normal sodium hydroxide digestion.

Polyester (Mersilene) net is a pliable material used for tissue reinforcement. Fixation is accomplished by fibroblastic proliferation into the interstices of the mesh.

Marlex mesh (knitted polypropylene) is a widely used biomaterial in the reinforcement of tissue at anastomotic sites and tissue defects. Earlier material designated as Marlex was high-density polyethylene, unlike the current

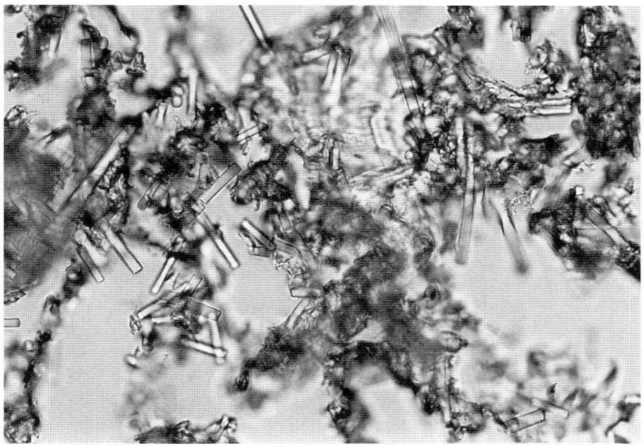

Fig. 4.5. Teflon, acute reaction. Rod-like crystals of injected Proplast (Teflon fluorocarbon polymer with carbon fibers) are present, with neutrophilic cellular reaction.

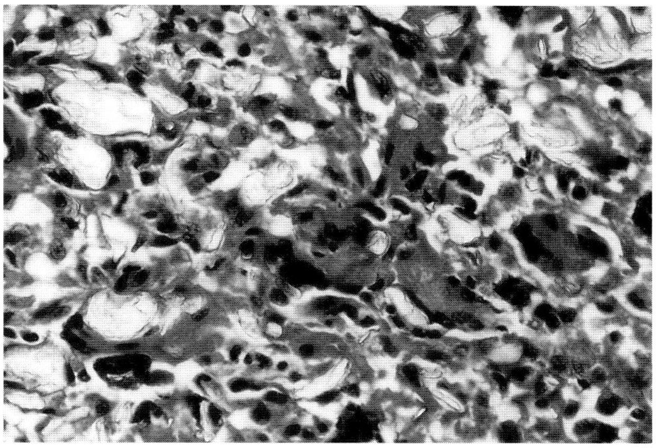

Fig. 4.6. Teflon granuloma. Foreign body giant cell reaction to Teflon. The Teflon appears as irregular refractile crystals.

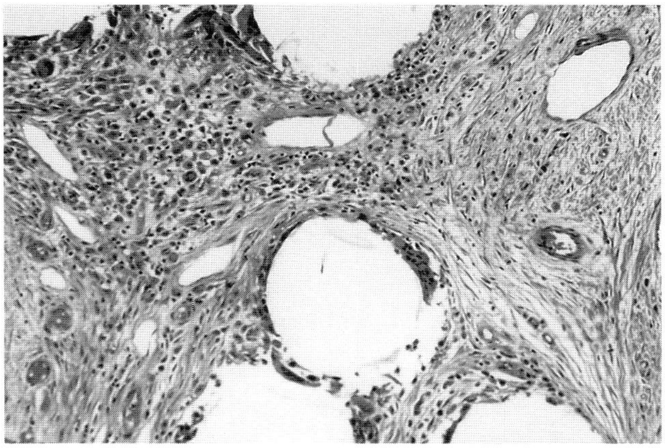

Fig. 4.7. Marlex mesh. The mesh is composed of multiple oval to round clear fibers, inducing a chronic inflammatory foreign body response and fibrosis.

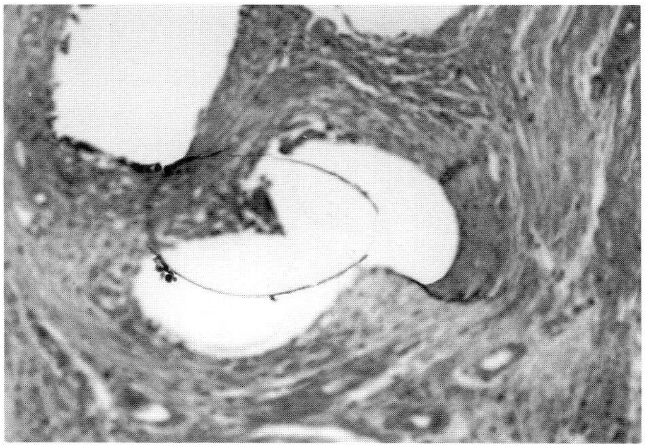

Fig. 4.8. Marlex mesh. High power demonstrates clear fibers, out of the plane of focus of the tissue.

low-density polypropylene material, which is more rigid, has a much longer flex life, and is more easily sterilized. Grossly, unincorporated Marlex mesh appears as sheets of clear plastic mesh. The process of incorporation of Marlex mesh into surrounding tissues is similar to that described for Dacron grafts. Microscopically, Marlex appears as round to oval clear fibers, which are highly birefringent.

Polyvinyl alcohol that has been crosslinked with formaldehyde (Ivalon) was commonly used as a surgical sponge and reconstructive material in the past. Some of its varied uses include tracheal reconstruction, hernia repairs, cardiac repairs, suture reinforcements, mammary augmentation, and even as artificial skin. The material has largely been replaced by silicones and other biomaterials, but is still found occasionally in tissue specimens from older people. Microscopically, Ivalon has sharply angular polygonal profiles and a slightly refractile gray–light brown appearance. After prolonged periods of time, the material may appear light blue and bubbly. The cellular response includes histiocytes, giant cells, and fibroblasts.

Silicone (polydimethylsiloxane) is a widely used biomaterial in medical devices. Its form is dependent upon the length of polymer chains and degree of crosslinking, ranging from fluid to a solid with properties similar to those of rubber. Differing pathologic reactions are seen with fluid (oils and gels) and solid forms of silicone.

Silicone rubber can be molded into a variety of shapes. It is commonly used in various prostheses for organ reconstruction, including eyes, ears, face, genitalia, and musculoskeletal parts. It is also fashioned into catheters and tubes of various types for surgical and medical applications. Probably the best known form of silicone prostheses is the silicone breast implant.

Early testing and reports about silicone found it to be one of the most biocompatible substances available, with no known physiologic harmful effects. However, more recently, numerous local and systemic effects of silicone have been described. Local reactions include infection, loosening, breakage, giant cell reaction, synovitis, osteolysis, erosion, and migration through soft tissues and skin. Silicone gel can be found in areas distant from the primary implantation site. Migration can be via soft tissues, lymphatics, and vessels. Patients undergoing hemodialysis and vascular procedures are at particular risk for hematogenous spread and embolization. Systemic complications that have been described include fever, malaise, delirium, acute pneumonitis, respiratory failure, renal failure, granulomatous hepatitis, lymphadenopathy, idiopathic thrombocytopenic purpura, and collagen vascular diseases. However, there is debate as to the whether silicone actually causes these diseases.

Silicone liquid has been injected into subcutaneous sites in plastic surgery procedures, especially into the breast. The U.S. Food and Drug Administration curbed the use of liquid silicone after recognition of many local reactions. Attempts to limit the local complications include placing silicone gel within bags for breast implants and adding vegetable oils and fatty acids to induce a scarring reaction to prevent the migration of silicone from the site of injection. The capsule may be smooth or textured, composed of either pure silicone or polyester/polyurethane foam covered silicone. Cellular response depends upon the composition of the capsule as well as the internal contents, mechanical forces, extent of leakage, and host response. Osmic acid, bromine silver, or phospholipid will stain vegetable oils (unsaturated fatty acids) that

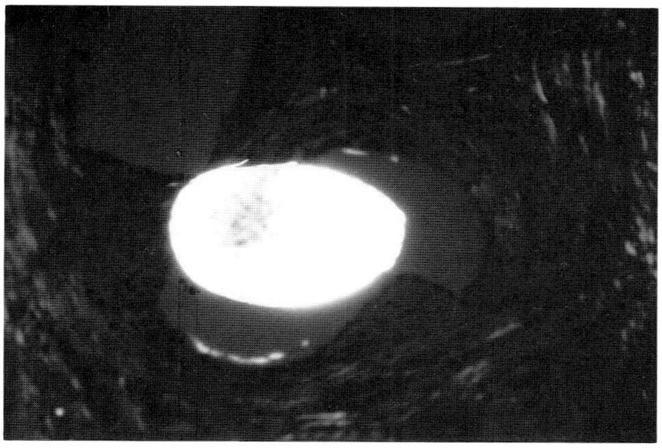

Fig. 4.9. Marlex mesh. Polarized view of the previous section.

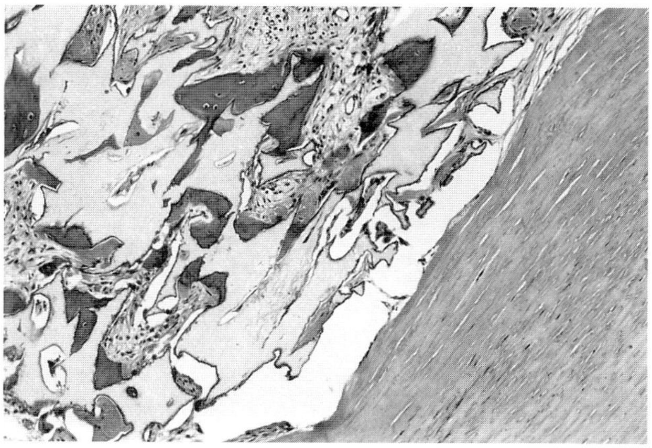

Fig. 4.10. Ivalon vascular graft material, which was in place for over 20 yr. The wall of the vessel is seen on the right side with irregular, slightly bubbly material. Dystrophic bone formation is seen accompanying the lesion.

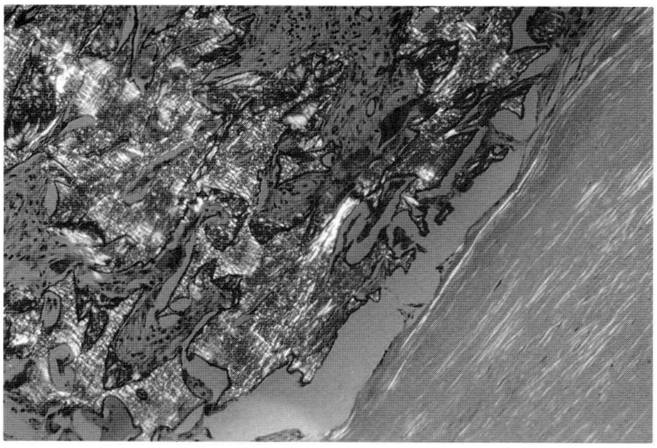

Fig. 4.11. Ivalon, polarized view of previous slide.

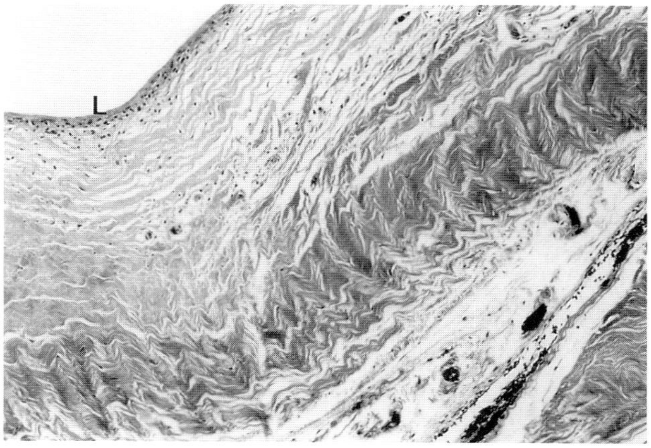

Fig. 4.12. Capsule of breast implant with smooth surface. Note that the capsule is composed of dense fibrous tissue and a synovium-like lining (L).

are added as adulterants. The fibrous capsule formed around silicone bags does not completely prevent leakage or slight fragmentation due to wear (known as the "bleed"). Recently, the use of silicone gel breast implants within bags has been halted due to questions about systemic complications. They have been replaced by less durable saline implants, which still are composed of solid silicone bags, but with saline contents.

Grossly, silicone appears as a liquid, a clear gel within bags (breast implants) or as a pliable solid material. Microscopically, liquid silicone is dissolved during routine processing and is recognized only by large empty vacuoles and its cellular reaction. Sheets of foamy macrophages make up the predominant cellular response to silicone oils. Gels induce the formation of sheets of foamy macrophages with scattered giant cells. Solid silicone appears as clear colorless refractile sheets; added materials often appear as polarizable granules. The response to solid silicone rubber is a mixed macrophage and giant cell reaction with granular and or smooth polyhedral fragments of clear refractile, nonbirefringent material. A fibrous capsule is usually formed to silicone bags, either lined by a smooth synovium-like lining, or a more undulating lining, depending upon the surface characteristics of the silicone bag. Textured silicone bags induce a knobby fibrous lining.

At times, a breast biopsy is performed for mammographic abnormalities in a patient with an implant, but no history is given to the pathologist. Microscopically, the scarring reaction and membrane lining simulate fat necrosis. However, there is typically a lack of true necrosis. The cyst that is formed with chronic fat necrosis is usually much smaller than an implant space. The spaces left by the silicone are more variable and often larger than those seen in fat necrosis.

LINES AND CATHETERS

Most lines and catheters in use today are made up of these substances: latex rubber, silicone, polyethylene, polypropylene, polytetrafluoroethylene, polyurethane, and polyvinyl chloride. The appearances of silicone, polypropylene, and polytetrafluoroethylene are described elsewhere in this chapter, since these substances are better known for their utilization in other medical applications.

Latex rubber is most commonly encountered as drainage tubes (Penrose), urinary catheters (Foley) or in the balloon portions of catheters. Latex is seen as yellow to clear sheets of soft, easily folded material. Typically, there are internal small, refractile golden granules.

Polyethylene tubing has diverse applications, such as in glaucoma, paranasal sinuses, middle ear vents, tear ducts, and prosthetic vas deferens. Polypropylene, which is easier to sterilize, is now used in many of these applications. Microscopically, polyethylene appears as clear sheets, often in geometric shapes. The edges of the material appear denser than the center, and only the edges are polarizable.

Polyvinyl chloride comes in a range of flexibilities, from rigid to pliable. It is used for chest tubes, intravenous tubes and bags, thermodilution catheters, among other applications. Microscopically, polyvinyl chloride is similar to

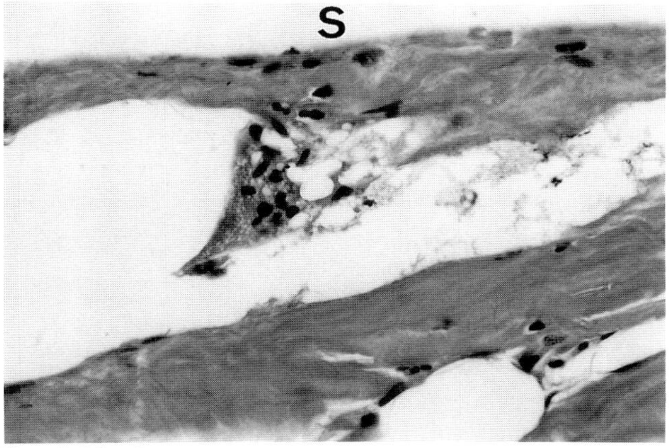

Fig. 4.13. Capsule of silicone breast implant. The surface of the implant was smooth, corresponding to this smooth fibrous wall (S). A multinucleated giant cell and a few histiocytes are seen in the stroma containing vacuolated silicone material.

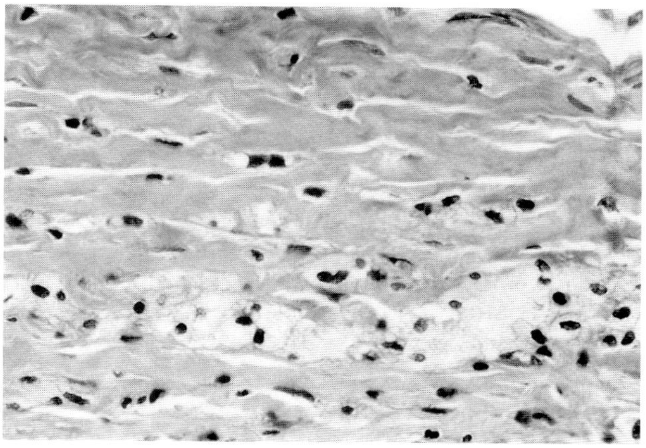

Fig. 4.14. Fibrous capsule of silicone breast implant, which was clinically intact. Note the numerous histiocytes containing fine vacuoles (the "bleed").

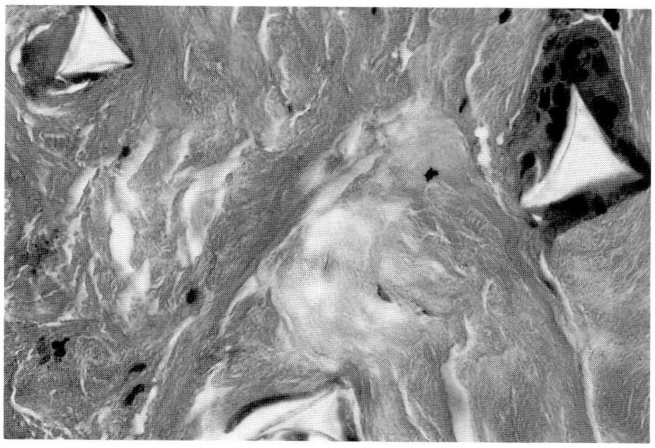

Fig. 4.15. Ruptured breast implant. Fibrous reaction at edge of implant contains clear triangular material within foreign body giant cells from polyurethane cover of implant.

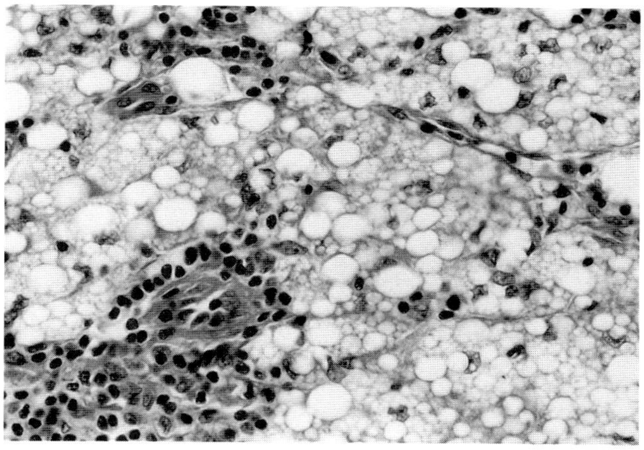

Fig. 4.16. Silicone breast implant leakage, axillary lymph node. Histiocytes in medullary sinuses are full of rounded vacuoles of varying sizes. The silicone is removed during processing.

other medical grade plastics, appearing as clear sheets with internal refractile, closely packed small golden granules.

Polyurethane refers to a family of long chain polymers containing diisocyante and polyol. The earlier compounds were quite biodegradable, but additives have improved their resistance to breakdown. Its decomposition products include 2,4-toluene diamine (TDA), which has been shown to be carcinogenic in laboratory animals, but not in humans. Besides lines and catheters, polyurethane covers have been used for breast implants, as well as for insulation for intravenous pacemaker leads.

SCLEROSING AGENTS

Silica was popularly used as a sclerosing agent 30–50 y ago for the therapy of inguinal hernias. Although not in current usage, inguinal nodules are still sometimes excised because of the florid fibrohistiocytic reaction, which may increase over time.

SUTURE MATERIAL

During any surgical procedure, suture is almost inevitably utilized. Depending upon use and needed strength, the size and type of suture varies. The histologic appearance of the suture depends upon its composition, configuration, size, and cellular reaction. Sutures may be composed of metal, naturally occurring substances, or synthetic compounds. The configuration of sutures is either as a monofilament (single cross-sectional view on a slide) or multifilament (multiple thread-like pieces on cross section). Multifilamentous sutures may be either twisted or braided together. Braided sutures are more prone to bacterial infection because bacteria may be trapped in interstices. Monofilament, synthetic sutures are more commonly used in nonsterile sites. The typically utilized size range is from 0 to 6–0 (the greater the 0–#, the thinner the suture), although sutures are manufactured in a greater range of sizes.

Initial tissue reaction is similar for all suture types during the first week after placement, assuming similar technique, tissue type, and lack of infection. Chronic reactions differ, depending upon the physical–chemical properties of the suture material. Sutures may be divided into two groups: (1) absorbable, those sutures that elicit an inflammatory response that breaks up the sutures and eventually destroys them; and (2) nonabsorbable, those sutures that remain more or less intact, but may be walled off by fibrous tissue and inflammatory cells. In general, synthetic materials elicit less of an inflammatory reaction than naturally occurring ones.

Absorbable sutures (Table 4.1) are used in sites that need the suture to approximate tissue edges until tissue repair takes place. They are preferred in buried, subcutaneous or mucosal sites. Placement of sutures in sites in which the sutures are not easily removed decreases the possibility of a longstanding suture acting as a nidus of infection.

Catgut is a monofilamentous suture composed of collagen derived from cattle flexor tendons or from intestines of sheep (submucosa) or cattle (serosa). Usual sites of application include perineal closures and subcutaneous vascular ties. Grossly, catgut is beige, slightly rough. Microscopically, catgut appears as a pink large round monofilament with an irregular interior. It is slightly

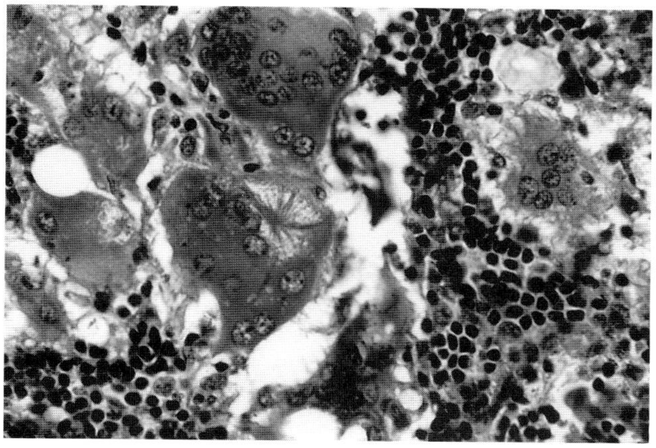

Fig. 4.17. Giant cell reaction to silicone in lymph node, with asteroid bodies.

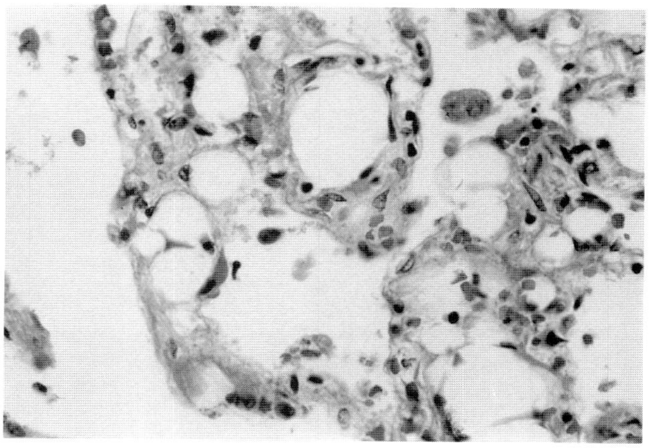

Fig. 4.18. Silicone embolus in lung, due to liquid silicone injection. Round extracellular spaces in alveolar walls are present.

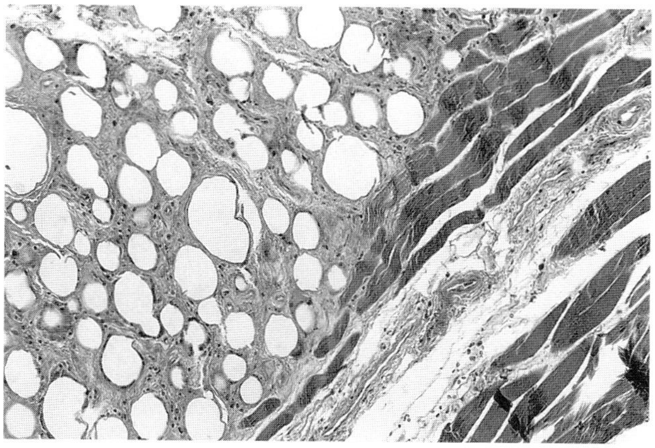

Fig. 4.19. Silicone in skeletal muscle. Patient had a leaking breast implant. The material is extracellular, making rounded spaces.

Fig. 4.20. Rubber. Light golden colored transparent sheets with numerous refractile dark granules.

Table 4.1. Absorbable Sutures

	Color (Gross)	Color (Micro, H&E)	Configuration
Catgut (± chromic)	beige	pink	monofilament
Polydioxanone (PDS)	beige or violet	clear	monofilament
Polyglycolic acid (Dexon)	beige	clear	braided, multifilament
Polyglactic acid (Vicryl)	beige or violet	clear or violet-blue	braided, multifilament
Polyglyconate (Maxon)	green-clear	clear	monofilament

refractile and polarizable. Absorption of catgut is through the process of phagocytosis and proteolysis. Plain catgut requires approximately 10 days for absorption. Chromium treatment of catgut doubles the absorption period to an average of 20 days. The tissue reaction is of the foreign body type and consists of a connective tissue capsule, histiocytes, lymphocytes, and capillary formation. Absorption is not always complete, and the previous suture site is typically marked by collection of monocytes with brown, foamy cytoplasm.

Polyglycolic acid (Dexon) and polyglactic acid (Vicryl) are synthetic, absorbable, braided sutures. They are routinely utilized in muscle, fascia, capsule, tendon, and subcutaneous closures. The gross appearance is of a light tan to golden multifilamentous suture, although dye may be added to give Vicryl a violet color. The cellular reaction is minimal because the sutures contain no antigens, collagen, or pyrogens. Typically, there are mononuclear cells in the vicinity of implanted sutures, with absorption due to hydrolysis of ester bonds. Complete absorption of sutures in 2–3 months is followed by disappearance of infiltrating cellular elements.

Polydioxanone (PDS) is a monofilament synthetic suture, which is absorbed by hydrolysis after a prolonged interval and has a high tensile strength. It can also be molded into clips and staples for flexible surgical use. Grossly, the suture is relatively stiff and either tan (undyed) or violet (dyed). The tissue reaction to PDS is milder than to most other absorbable sutures.

Maxon (polyglyconate monofilament) appears similar to PDS.

Nonabsorbable sutures (Table 4.2) are used in sites that depend upon permanent tissue bonds, such as heart valves and vascular grafts. They are also commonly employed in superficial sites, in which the suture is removed after initial tissue repair.

A low carbon iron alloy is used in the manufacture of stainless steel **wire.** It comes in either mono- or multifilament forms. Orthopedic surgery constitutes its most frequent use, in tissues such as ligaments, tendon, and bone. The widespread application of computed tomography and nuclear magnetic resonance imaging techniques has made these sutures less desirable because of the artifacts and/or movement induced by metal in the images. In addition, metallic sutures are known to cut through gloves, and increase the probability of the transmission of infectious diseases, such as hepatitis or the AIDS virus.

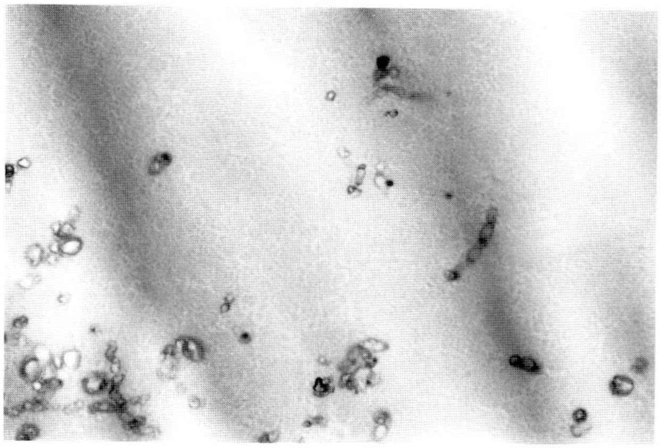

Fig. 4.21. Foley catheter fragment that was broken off and retained in the bladder. There are fungal hyphae and calcium oxalate crystals present, which are growing within this matrix.

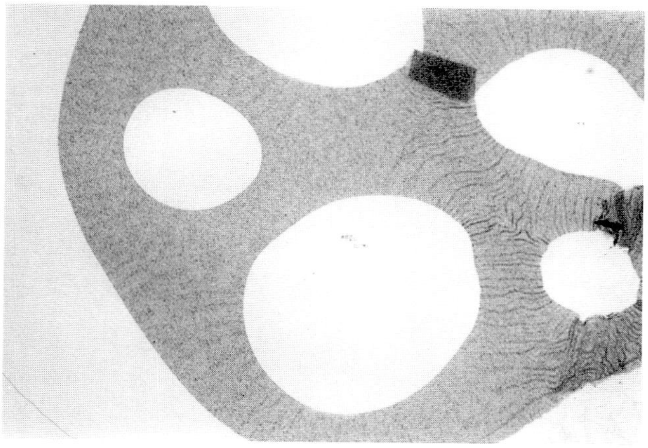

Fig. 4.22. Swan-Ganz catheter. Five round lumens are present within a granular matrix.

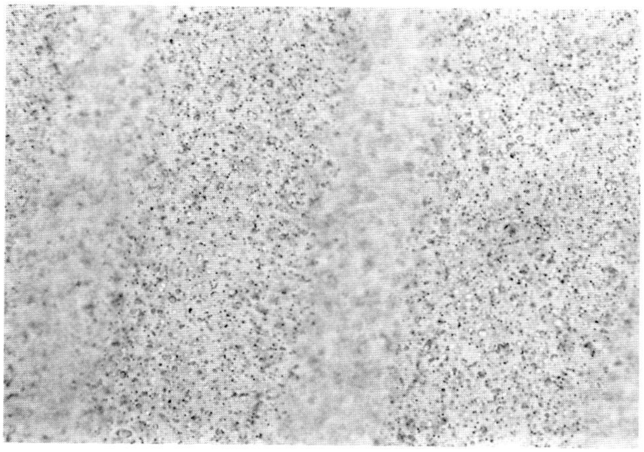

Fig. 4.23. Swan-Ganz catheter, higher power. The catheter matrix contains numerous black-gray granules of varying sizes. Only portions of the specimen focus on any one plane due to folding during sectioning.

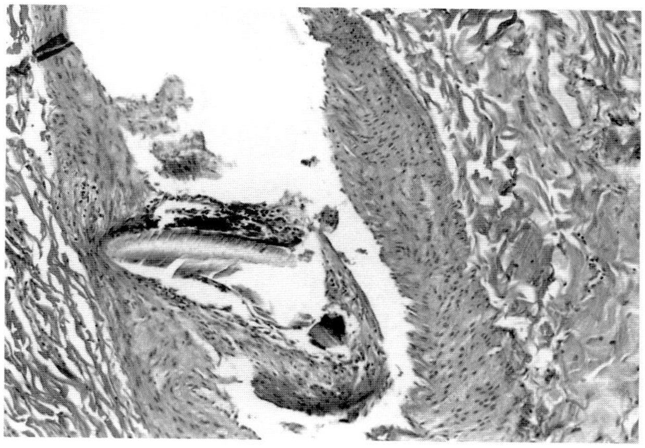

Fig. 4.24. Catheter fragment embedded in a pulmonary vein, causing a foreign body giant cell reaction.

Table 4.2. Nonabsorbable Sutures

	Color (Gross)	Color (Micro)	Configuration
Wire	silver	black	monofilament or multifilament
Silk	black	gray	multifilament
Cotton	variable	clear	multifilament
Polypropylene (Prolene)	clear or blue	clear or blue	monofilament
Polyester	variable	clear	monofilament or multifilament
Nylon	clear, black, or green	clear, gray, or blue	monofilament or multifilament

Metal sutures are normally removed from tissue prior to processing; therefore only the empty space and its mononuclear cellular reaction are observable routinely.

Silk is a braided, naturally occurring protein suture. Grossly, it appears to be a pliable black thread. It is classified as a nonabsorbable suture, but in fact, does degrade after a variable period. The microscopic appearances of silk suture is of gray, multiple sharply and irregularly angulated fibers, of variable sizes. The cellular reaction to silk is usually marked, including a fibrous capsule, with an underlying layer of histiocytes, giant cells, and lymphocytes. Capillaries may sometimes be prominent.

Cotton is similar to silk in its texture, reactivity, and braided configuration. Microscopically cotton fibers appear to be clear to blue oval or U-shaped rings. It is quite refractile and polarizable.

Polypropylene (Prolene) is an extremely smooth monofilamentous synthetic suture. It is available in clear or blue-dyed forms. Its ease of removal and high strength make it useful in cutaneous sites. The synthetic monofilament is also widely applied in infected closures and microvascular surgery. Microscopically, the suture appears to be a round clear monofilament with numerous minute blue granules.

Polyester (Mersilene, Tevdek, Tricron, Ethibond, Novafil) is extremely strong, but requires more knots to stabilize the suture than most other suture types. It is characteristically used in sterile fascial closures. Polyester sutures are usually braided in configuration and come in a variety of forms, depending upon coating. Plain polyester suture (Mersilene) tends to cut tissue as it is pulled through, so Teflon (Tevdek), silicone (Tricron), and polybutylate (Ethibond) have been used to coat polyester to lessen this effect. A monofilamentous form is also available as Novafil, which appears to be smoother and somewhat stiffer than the braided forms.

Nylon is a synthetic polyamide polymer, in either monofilament (Ethilon) or multifilament forms. Most commonly, it is used in cutaneous surgery because of its low cellular reactivity, therefore causing minimal scarring. Grossly, nylon appears as a black, green or clear smooth suture. Microscopically nylon appears as a clear substance with golden color. It stains by

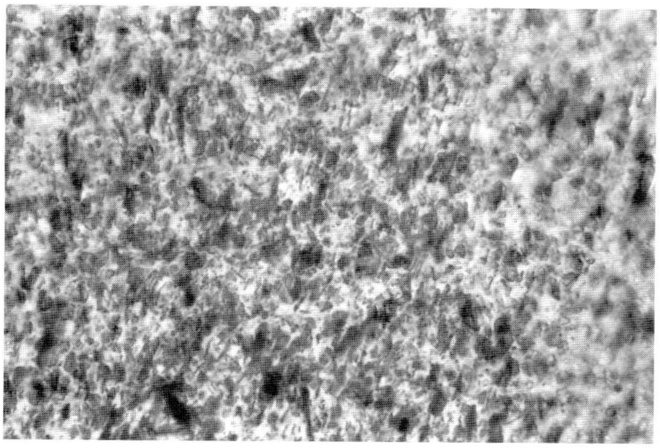

Fig. 4.25. Stent, ureteral. Numerous dark refractile granules, some in clumps.

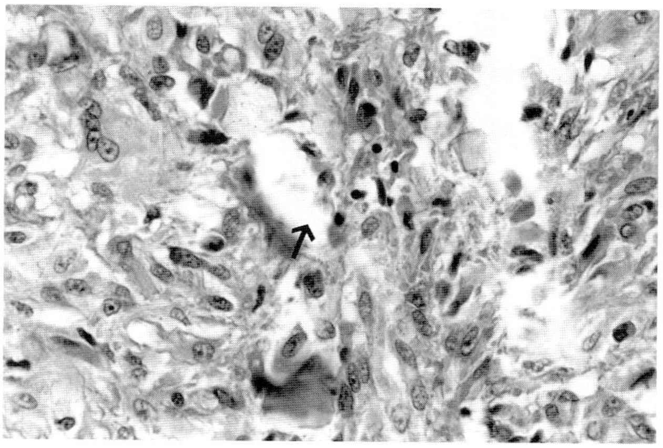

Fig. 4.26. Silica, hernia sac. This hernia sac had been injected with silica, which was used as a sclerosing agent, several decades prior. There is a reactive fibrohistiocytic response with poorly visualized intra- and extracellular silica crystals (*arrow*).

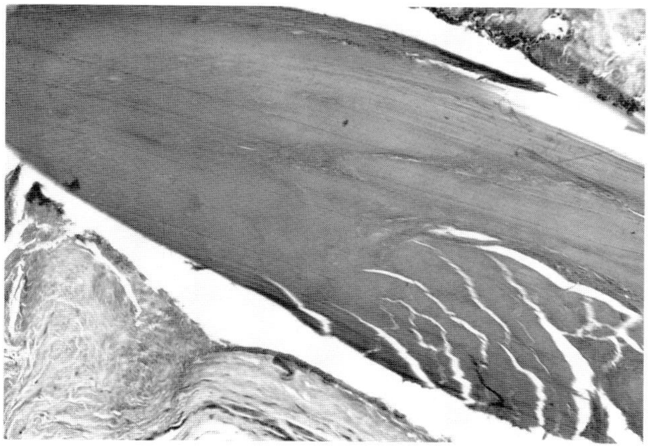

Fig. 4.27. Catgut suture. Large eosinophilic monofilamentous suture that has linear parallel streaks.

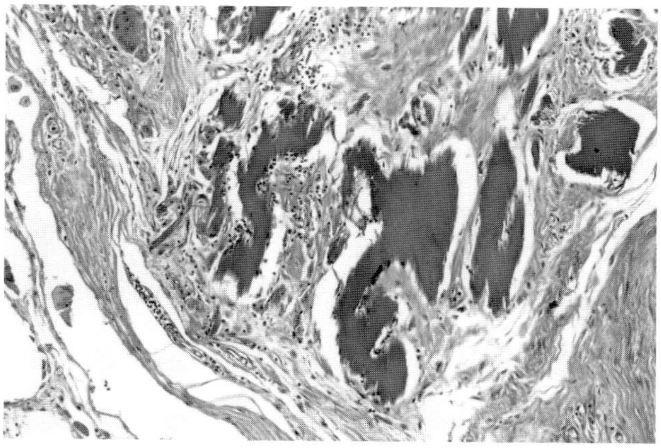

Fig. 4.28. Catgut suture. 7 months after surgery. The suture is being broken down and a chronic inflammatory reaction is present. The suture material often fragments when cut on the microtome.

anthraquinone and has a positive birefringence. Degradation takes place in about 2 yrs.

Nonabsorbable surgical clips may be composed of stainless steel, titanium, tantalum, or nylon. These materials are extremely hard and will not typically be seen in histologic sections. **Absorbable surgical clips** are composed of polydioxane, which appears as described above under sutures.

PACKING, SPONGES, SWABS, GLOVE RESIDUE

These products are primarily composed of cotton, cellulose, and collagen, but may also include polyester, polyethylene, polyurethane, and other products.

Cotton is the primary component of cotton drapes, balls, and pads. Cotton products allow the absorption of fluid into the spaces between fibers. Grossly, cotton is a soft white fiber. Microscopically, each individual fiber is seen as oval to U-shaped rings. These fibers appear clear to pale blue and are both refractile and polarizable. Blood and other fluids may appear in between fibers. If a cotton pad is accidentally left in vivo during a surgical procedure, a fibroinflammatory reaction ensues.

Telfa pads are white soft pads, composed of polyurethane and cotton or rayon. The surface of the telfa pad is shiny and smooth, allowing relatively little tissue to adhere. Microscopically, the telfa pad appears as round fibers with minute black particles.

Rayon is a processed cotton fiber. Microscopically, rayon fibers are light blue on hematoxylin–eosin (H&E) and contain minute brown granules. They are birefringent on polarized light microscopy.

Packing materials include cellulose, calcium alginate, collagen, gelatin, and rayon/acrylic binders. *Surgicell* is a regenerated cellulose/polyester compound. Microscopically, Surgicell is seen as long, irregular bands of pale violet material. *Calcium alginate* (Algoderm) is composed of broad blue strands of finely fibrillar material. *Collagen* (Mallitene) packing appears as irregular pink fibrils, which are weakly polarizable. *Gelatin* (*Gelfoam*) is characterized by anastomosing curvilinear, dense, homogeneous pink material.

Starch granules are commonly used to lubricate surgical gloves. These granules may incite a granulomatous foreign body reaction with numerous giant cells. Starch granules appear as grouped basophilic structures, 10–20 μm in size, in "Maltese cross" configurations. The granules stain positively with periodic acid–Schiff (PAS) and methenamine silver and are highly birefringent.

Talc particles have been used to lubricate gloves, and as an agent to cut drugs, both legal and illegal, since talc is relatively inert (see Chapter 8, Minerals and Metals).

Specimens may be placed on **paper or cardboard** after excision. These materials are composed of cellulose fibers in various configurations and are typically strongly anisotropic.

ARTIFICIAL JOINT IMPLANTS

Joint implants typically consist of a metallic articular surface, articulated with either a polyethylene or ceramic acetabular component, and supported by a metal framework attached to native bone. A glue composed of methyl

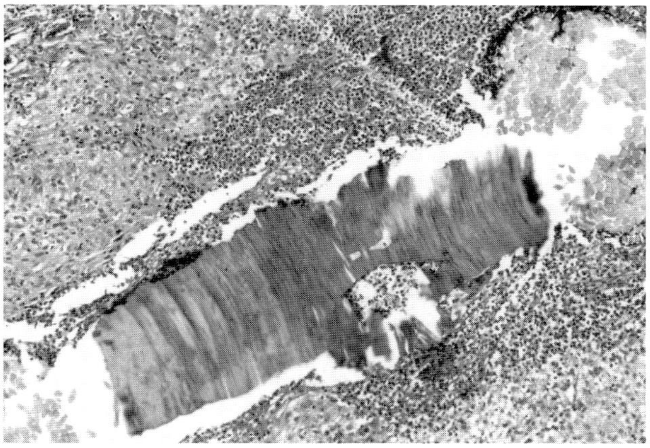

Fig. 4.29. Chromic suture, similar in microscopic appearance to regular catgut. A florid acute inflammatory response is present. An adjacent multifilament fiber is seen on the right.

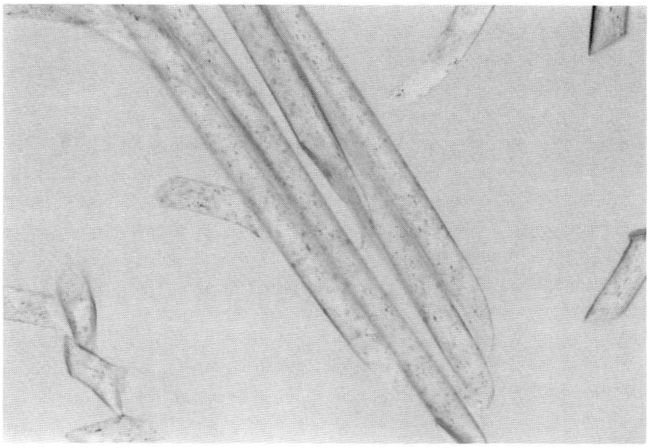

Fig. 4.30. Vicryl suture. Note the fine black granules within clear cylindrical fibers.

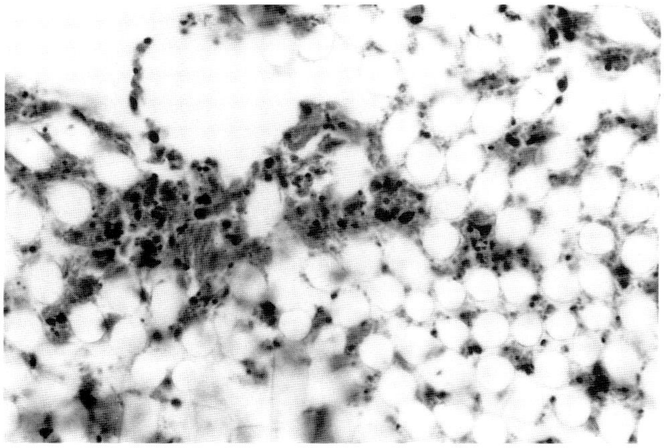

Fig. 4.31. Vicryl suture, 1 wk after surgery. Vicryl is a multifilamentous synthetic absorbable suture. Round clear fibers are seen in cross section, with an infiltrate of acute inflammatory cells.

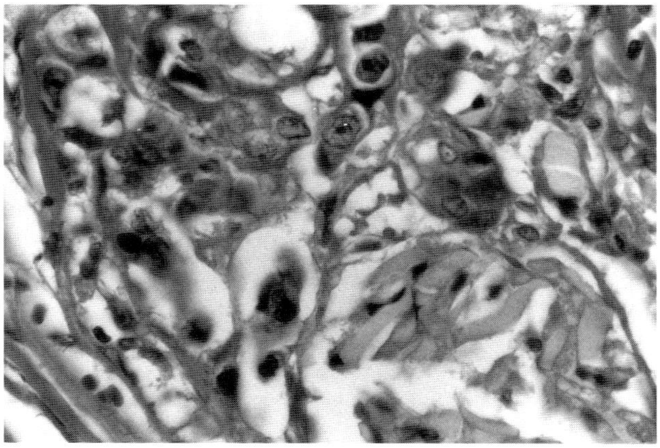

Fig. 4.32. Vicryl suture, 7 months after surgery. Note multiple synthetic fibers at varying angles. Inflammatory response at this time is chronic.

methacrylate fills the spaces between the bone, plastic and metal components of the joint. Methyl methacrylate begins as a liquid monomer, which polymerizes into soft mass when mixed with polymethyl methacrylate and is then usable as a cementing agent. Barium sulfate is added to the mixture for radiographic visibility. During the polymerization process, heat is produced and partial release of the monomer into the bloodstream is possible, with systemic complications described.

Upon initial implantation, the tissue response around the functioning prosthesis begins with necrosis due to surgical disruption of blood supply, heat of polymerization, and the local toxic effect of the monomer. After approximately a week, repair takes place, with granulation tissue formation and osteoclastic resorption of bone. This process of remodeling is completed within 2 y, with formation of a fibrous membrane between bone and cement. This fibrous membrane isolates the foreign material and also acts as biologic shock absorber to mechanical stress. Fibrocartilaginous metaplasia or osseous replacement may also occur.

If the joint implant fails, due to either infection or mechanical failure, the joint implant and its surrounding tissues may be removed and sent for pathologic examination. If the failure was caused by infection, signs of inflammation are present. Organisms may or may not be identified on special stains. In a purely mechanical failure, hyperplasia of the synovium is usually seen. The adjacent tissue shows evidence of wear debris, with a foreign body granulomatous reaction. This wear debris is composed of any combination of the elements of the joint implant: metal, polyethylene, ceramic, or methyl methacrylate.

Metallic debris may induce osteolysis, thus loosening of the implant. A significant amount of metal deposition causes a gross appearance of gray to black synovium. On microscopic examination, histiocytes are seen containing small, irregular black fragments, usually 1–3 μm in size. Under polarized light, the particle edges are visualized, particularly around titanium implants. Material may also accumulate in local draining lymph nodes and a granulomatous response may occur. Not only can metallic wear products be found, but metals may corrode, with products that have cytotoxic, hypersensitivity, and possibly even carcinogenic effects.

Polyethylene, when grossly visualized on joint implants, is a white firm uniform plastic substance on the metallic surface. Microscopically, fibrillar fragments measuring 10–20 μm within histiocytes and giant cells are seen under polarized light microscopy.

The adjacent methyl methacrylate displays a wide range in size, with some particles greater than 100 μm. It is dissolved during normal processing procedures, but residual polygonal shapes within giant cells are characteristic of methyl methacrylate. Finer particles may also be present in histiocytes. In addition, barium crystals remain and are visible as green-brown granules.

Another "glue" used as a tissue adhesive in wound healing is cyanoacrylate (n-butyl cyanoacrylate). Like methyl methacrylate, it typically leaches out during deparaffinization. It can be demonstrated by using petroleum ether to remove paraffin. Microscopically, cyanoacrylate appears as an amorphous, irregular material at the surface of wounds. Blood and chronic inflammatory cells may be incorporated within the material.

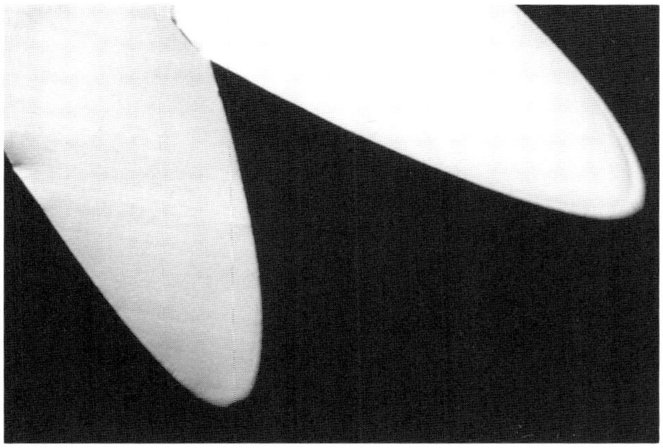

Fig. 4.33. PDS (polydioxanone) suture. PDS is a monofilamentous synthetic suture. It is much more easily visualized using polarized microscopy.

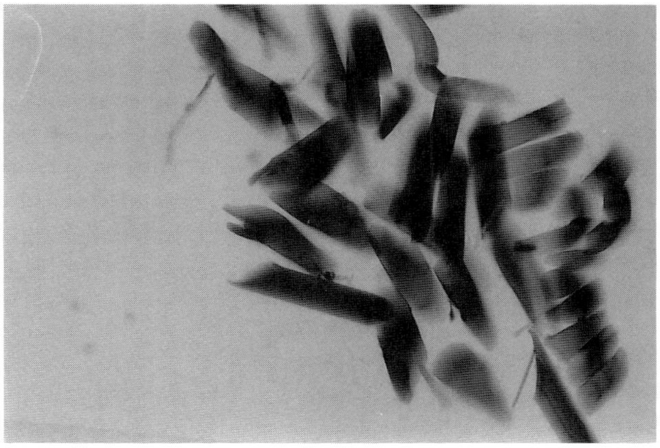

Fig. 4.34. Silk suture. Silk is a multifilament braided suture. Note bundle of fibers, some parallel to each other, others at angles to each other. On H&E stain, these fibers appear gray.

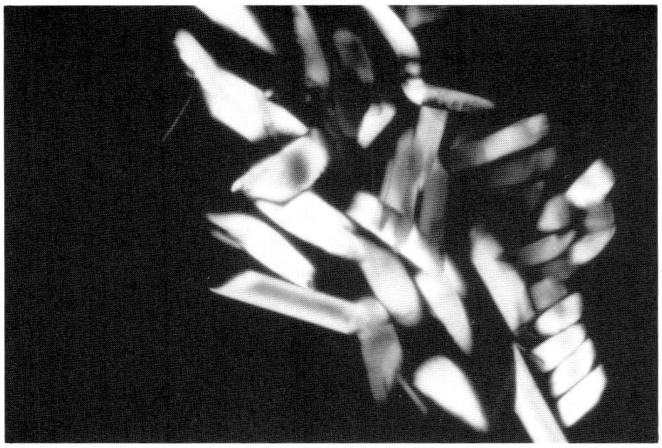

Fig. 4.35. Silk suture, polarized view. This view shows a cross section of silk, with each fiber appearing as polygonal shapes.

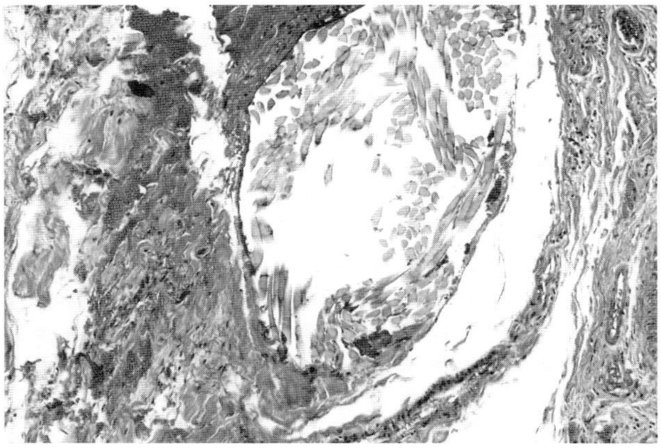

Fig. 4.36. Silk suture embedded in subcutaneous collagen. Note multifilamentous fibers, with slightly curved triangular or rectangular shapes, admixed with more elongated fibers.

The differential diagnosis of the giant cell reaction around joint spaces includes giant cell tumor of tendon sheath, aneurysmal bone cyst, pigmented villonodular tenosynovitis, rheumatoid arthritis, hyperparathyroidism, and granulomatous infections. All other entities are nonpolarizable and lack the characteristic polygonal spaces of joint wear debris.

BIBLIOGRAPHY

Bullough PG, DiCarlo EF, Hansraj KK, et al: Pathologic studies of total joint replacement. *Orthop Clin North Am* 19:611–625, 1988.

Craig PH, Williams JA, Davis KW, et al: A biologic comparison of polyglactin 910 and polyglycolic acid synthetic absorbable sutures. *Surg Obstet Gynecol* 141:1–10, 1975.

Gulati SM, Thusoo TK, Kakar A, et al: Comparative study of free omental, peritoneal, dacron velour, and marlex mesh reinforcement of large-bowel anastomosis. *Dis Col Rect* 25:517–521, 1982.

Hameed MR, Erlandson R, Rosen PP: Capsular synovial-like hyperplasia around mammary implants similar to detritic synovitis. *Am J Surg Pathol* 19:433–438, 1995.

Harboldt SL, Gumley GJ, Balogh K: Osteolysis after silicone arthroplasty. *Am J Clin Pathol* 98:594–597, 1992.

Hastings JC, Van Winkle W, Barker E, et al: Effect of suture materials on healing wounds of the stomach and colon. *Surg Gynecol Obstet* 140:701–707, 1975.

Hyman FN, Klontz KC, Tollefson L: Eating as a hazard to health: preventing, treating dental injuries caused by foreign objects in food. *JADA* 124:65–69, 1993.

Kasper CS: Histologic features of breast capsules reflect surface configuration and composition of silicone bag implants. *Am J Clin Pathol* 102:655–659, 1994.

Kepes JJ, Yarde WL: Visualization of injected embolic material (polyvinyl alcohol) in paraffin sections with Verhoeff-Van Gieson elastica stain. *Am J Surg Pathol* 19: 709–711, 1995.

Kossovsky N, Cole P, Zackson DA: Giant cell myocarditis associated with silicone. *Am J Clin Pathol* 93:148–152, 1990.

Leong ASY, Disney APS, Gove DW: Spallation and migration of silicone from blood-pump tubing in patients on hemodialysis. *N Engl J Med* 306:135–140, 1982.

Postlethwait RW, Willigan DA, Ulin AW: Human tissue reaction to sutures. *Ann Surg* 181:144–150, 1975.

Robinson MJ, Nestor M, Rywlin AM: Pulmonary granulomas secondary to embolic prosthetic valve material. *Hum Pathol* 12:759–762, 1981.

Sanz LE, Patterson JA, Kamath R, et al: Comparison of maxon suture with vicryl, chromic catgut, and PDS sutures in fascial closure in rats. *Obstet Gynecol* 71: 418–422, 1988.

Sato O, Tada Y, Takagi A: The biologic fate of dacron double velour vascular prosthesis. *Japan J Surg* 19:301–311, 1989.

Schoen FJ, Harasake H, Kim KM, et al: Biomaterial-associated calcification: pathology, mechanisms, and strategies for prevention. *J Biomed Mater Res: Applied Biomaterials* 22 A1:11–36, 1988.

Schoetz DJ, Coller JA, Veidenheimer MC: Closure of abdominal wounds with polydioxanone. *Arch Surg* 123:72–74, 1988.

Smit IB, Witte E, Brand R, et al: Tissue reaction to suture materials revisited: is there argument to change our views? *Eur Surg Res* 23:347–354, 1991.

Snyder CC: On the history of the suture. *Plast Reconst Surg* 58:401–406, 1976.

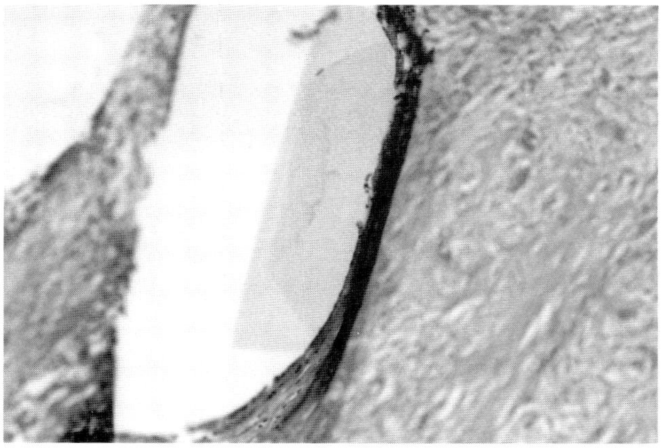

Fig. 4.37. Polypropylene (Prolene) suture. Prolene appears as a clear blue monofilamentous suture, which often folds during the process of cutting the block. Note the suture is carried out of its original space and appears in a different plane of focus from the remainder of the specimen.

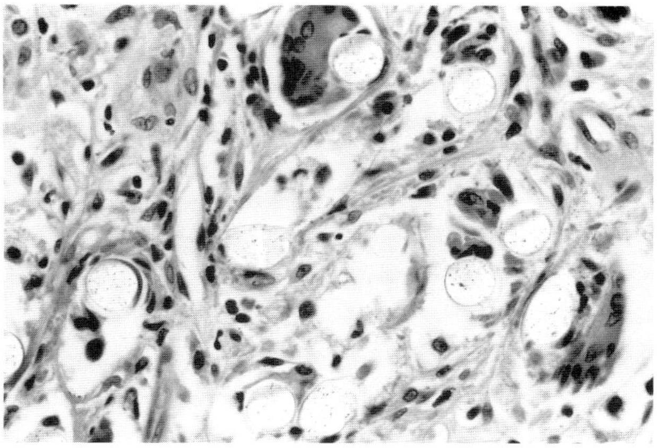

Fig. 4.38. Ethibond suture. Ethibond is an example of a polyester suture, which is multifilamentous, with fine black granules within the fibers.

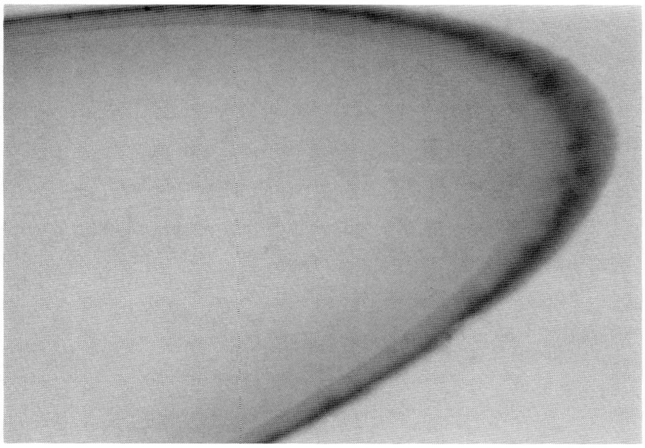

Fig. 4.39. Ethilon suture. Ethilon is a monofilamentous nylon suture.

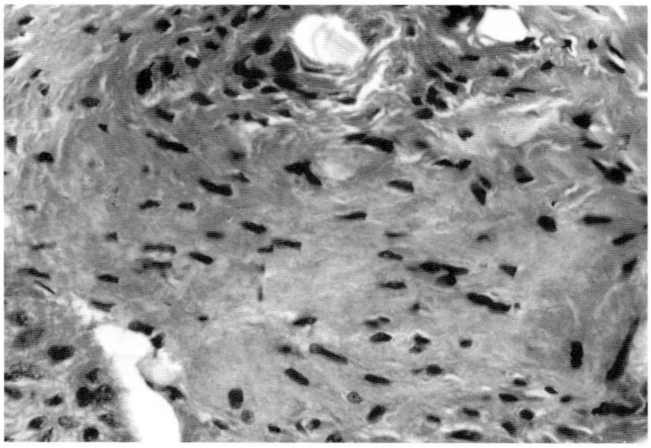

Fig. 4.40. Tricron suture. Tricron is a multifilamentous nylon suture. Note that a marked chronic reaction has occurred, with dense fibrous tissue surrounding the filaments.

Travis WD, Balogh K, Abraham JL: Silicone granulomas: report of three cases and review of the literature. *Hum Pathol* 16:19–27, 1985.

Tubbs RR, Picha GC, Levin HS, et al: Cotton emboli (cellulose II polymorph, "rayon") of the coronary arteries. *Hum Pathol* 11:76–80, 1980.

Van der Leij G, van Krimpen C: Impact of ovabloc intratubal polymer on the morphology of the fallopian tube. *Int J Gynecol Pathol* 14:167–173, 1995.

Walley VM, Stinson WA, Upton C, et al: Foreign materials found in the cardiovascular system after instrumentation or surgery. *Cardiovasc Pathol* 2:157–185, 1993.

Weiss SW, Enzinger FM, Johnson FB. Silica reaction simulating fibrous histiocytoma. *Cancer* 42:2738–2743, 1978.

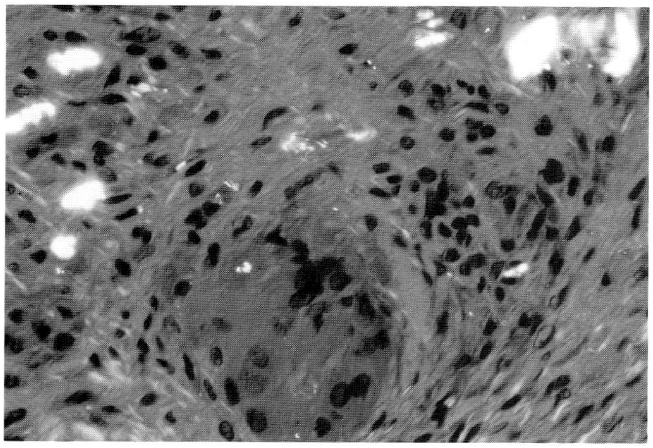

Fig. 4.41. Tricron suture, polarized light. More fragments of suture were present than could be appreciated by routine light microscopy.

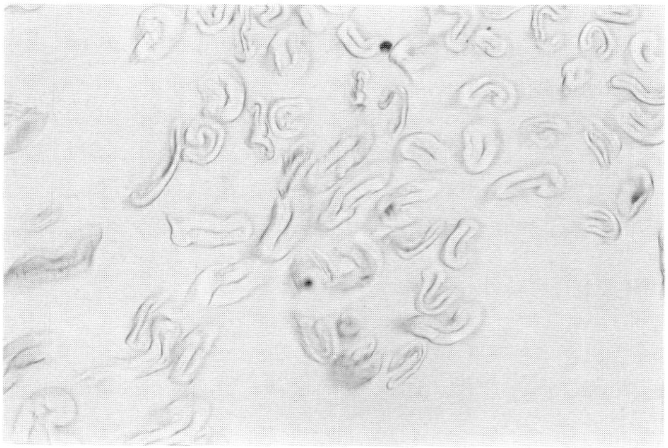

Fig. 4.42. Cotton suture. Cotton is composed of numerous transparent hollow discoid fibers, some of which are folded.

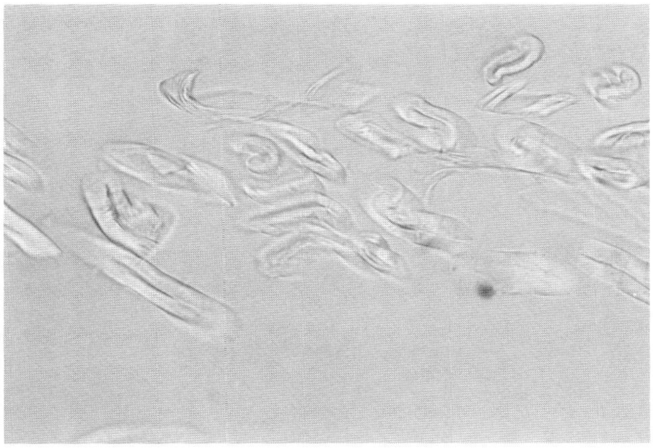

Fig. 4.43. Cotton gauze pad. Cotton fibers appear microscopically as clear hollow ovoid structures. The fibers of a gauze pad face multiple directions and are held together in parallel bands. The microscopic appearance is identical to that of cotton suture.

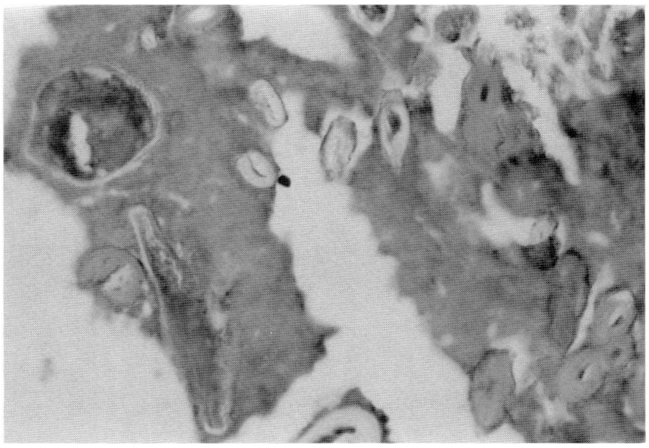

Fig. 4.44. Vaginal foreign body, removed by a gynecologist. There are numerous hollow oval clear structures (cotton) amid amorphous eosinophilic fibrin and bacteria.

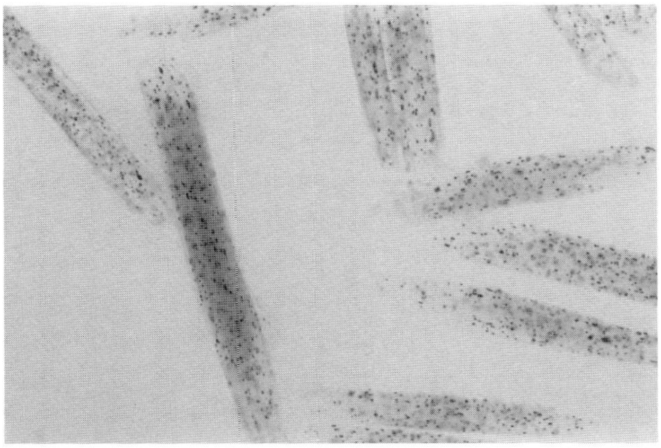

Fig. 4.45. Tampon fibers. Cylindrical fibers, with acute angular ends, showing numerous black internal granules (rayon).

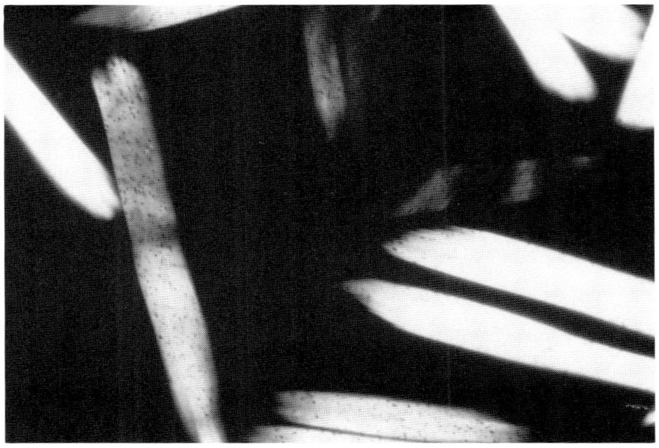

Fig. 4.46. Tampon fibers, polarized view. The fibers are strongly birefringent, but the internal black granules do not polarize.

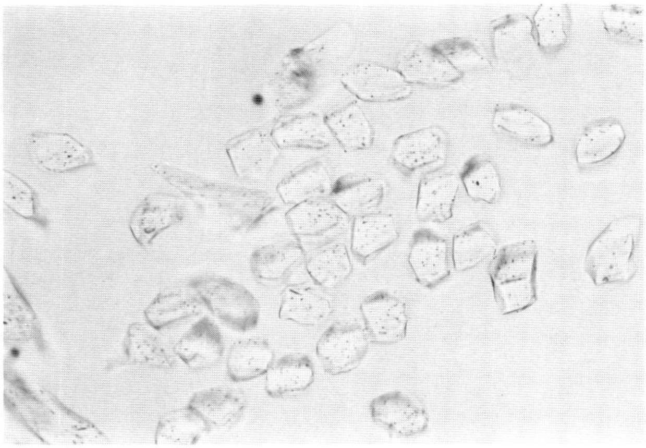

Fig. 4.47. Mask, polyester fibers. The material is composed of angular filaments in a loose tile-like arrangement. Each filament contains numerous black granules.

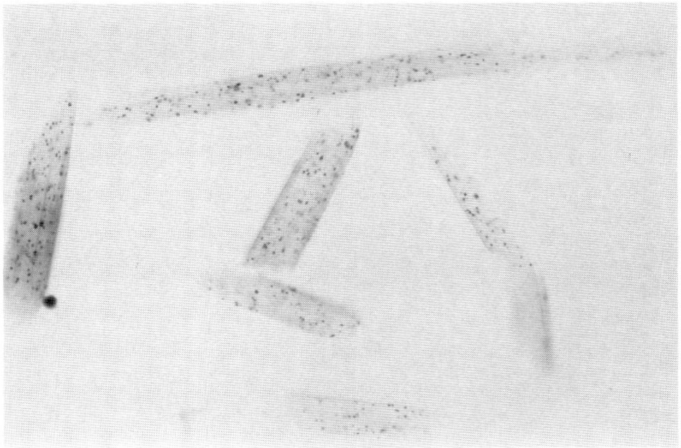

Fig. 4.48. Rayon in alcohol pad. Note the linear fibers with parallel edges and numerous refractile black particles within.

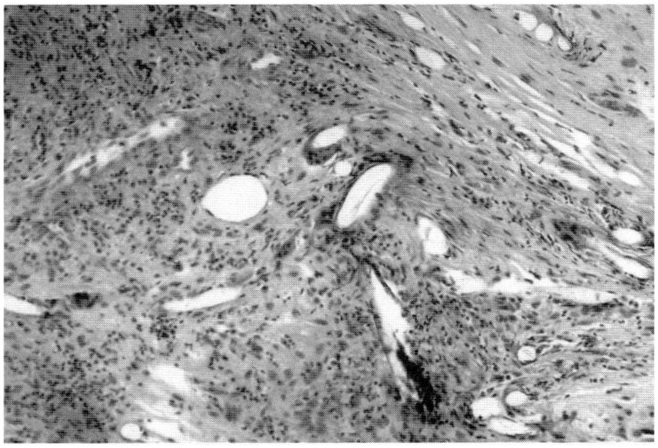

Fig. 4.49. Telfa pad left in peritoneal cavity. Round to oval clear fibers with minute black granules. There is a fibrous reaction and foreign body giant cells are seen engulfing the fibers.

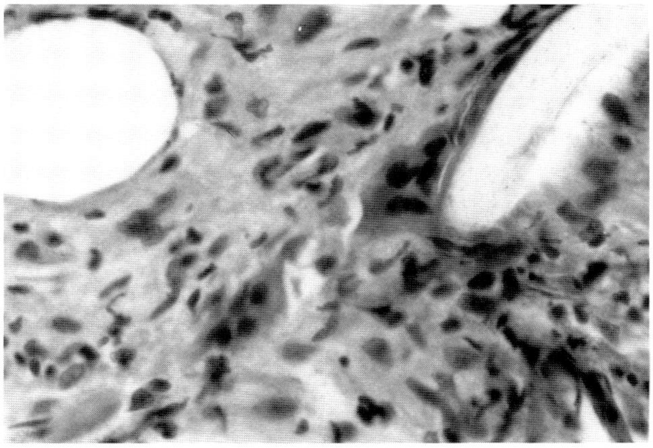

Fig. 4.50. Telfa pad, same as above, higher power. Note that the fiber (on the right) is in a slightly different plane of focus from the cells.

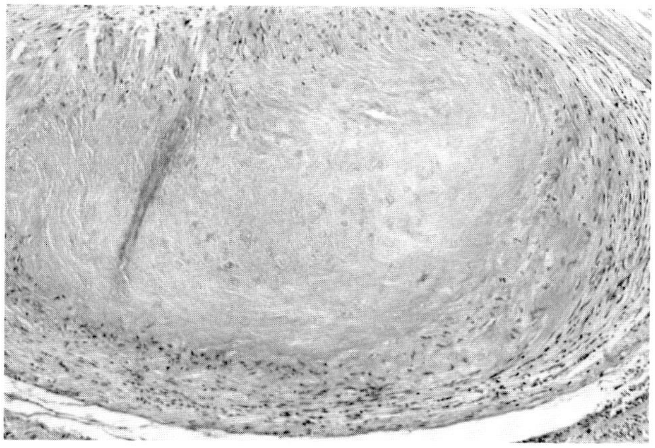

Fig. 4.51. Starch granuloma in peritoneal cavity, 5 months after abdominal surgery. Multiple white miliary particles were found upon reexploration surgery for continuing abdominal pain. A fibrous wall surrounds the granuloma, which contains refractile round clear particles, approximately the size of adjacent nuclei of inflammatory cells. These particles have a central black dot on H&E stain and are PAS-positive.

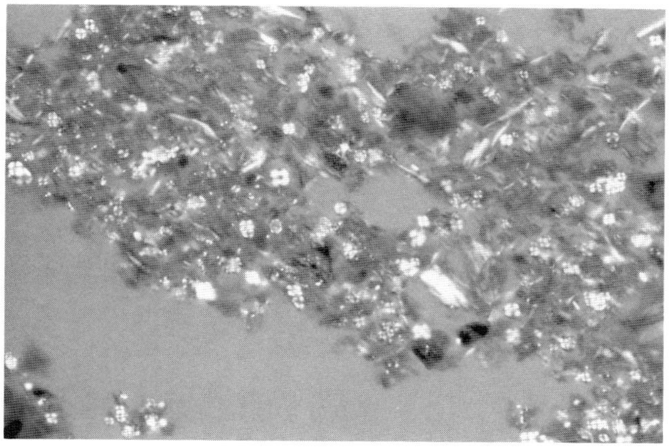

Fig. 4.52. Starch granuloma, higher power, polarized microscopy. The "Maltese cross" configuration of starch granules is characteristic.

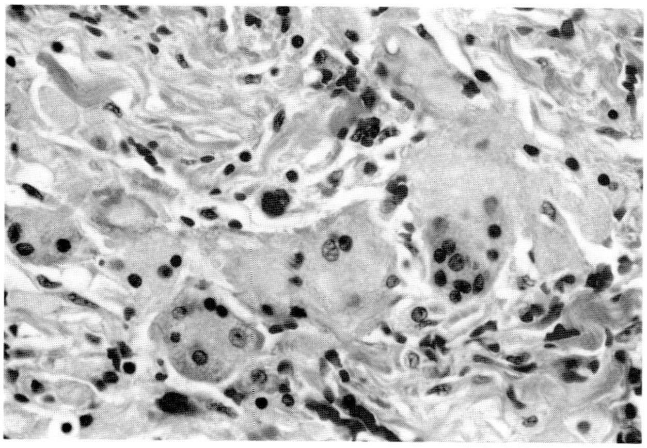

Fig. 4.53. Talc, inciting foreign body reaction. The plate-like crystals of talc are barely visible on routine light microscopy.

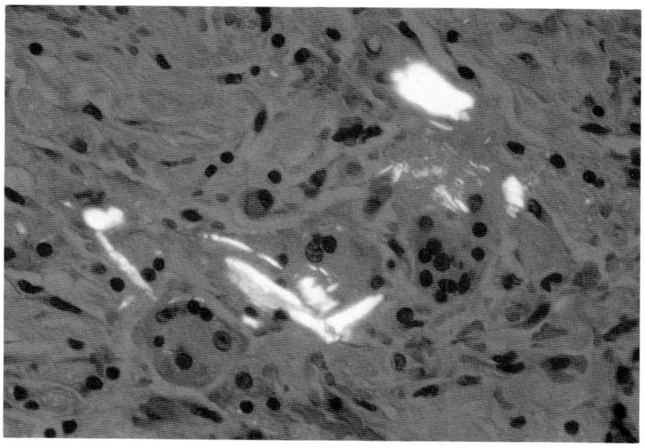

Fig. 4.54. Talc, polarized view. The fibers are markedly birefringent on polarized light microscopy.

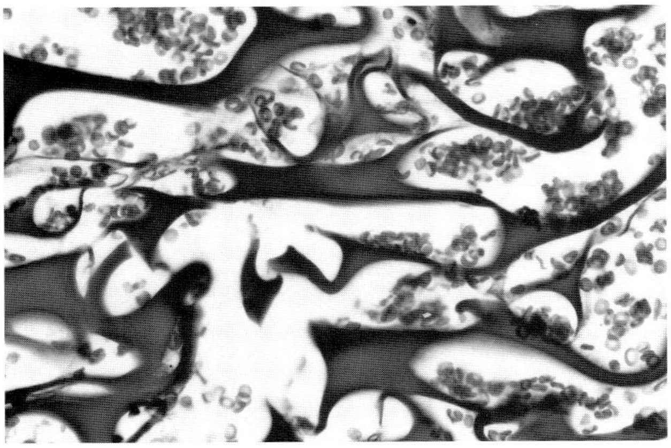

Fig. 4.55. Gelfoam, used in surgery for pituitary adenoma. The material is composed of anastomosing angulated dense pink material on H&E stain. Note that the spaces are filled with blood, since the Gelfoam has been used as a sponge.

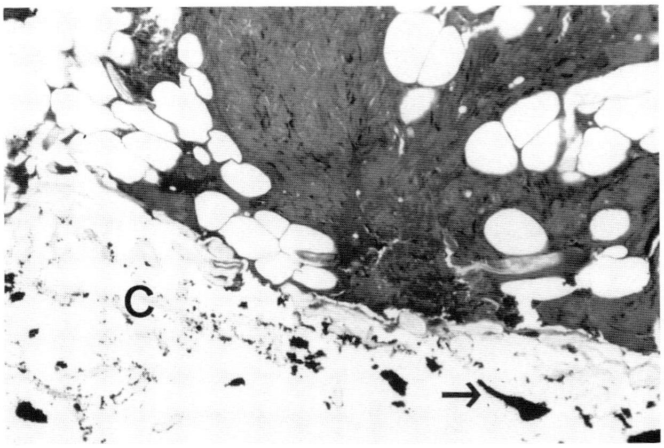

Fig. 4.56. Cardboard, at the edge of a tissue section. Tissue was hard to cut and shows folds. The cardboard (C) is composed of almost transparent fibers. Black material is graphite (*arrow*).

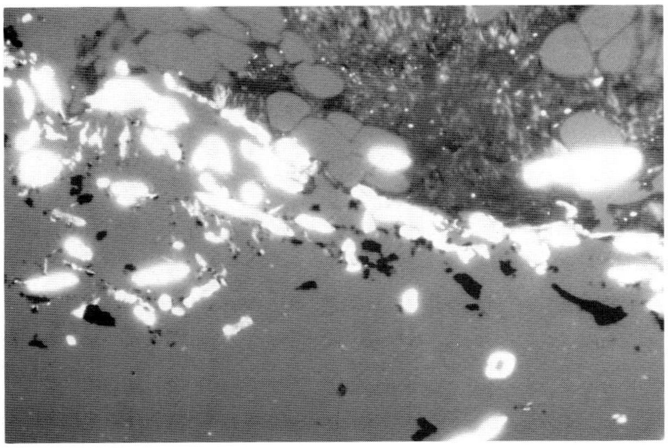

Fig. 4.57. Cardboard, with polarized light. Note variable fiber types including hollow oval configurations.

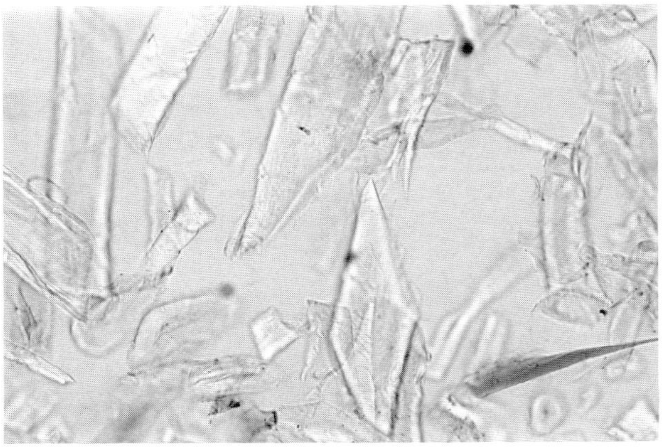

Fig. 4.58. Paper towel, which was underneath a specimen. The paper is made of cellulose fibers, in irregular angulated and oval shapes with parallel edges.

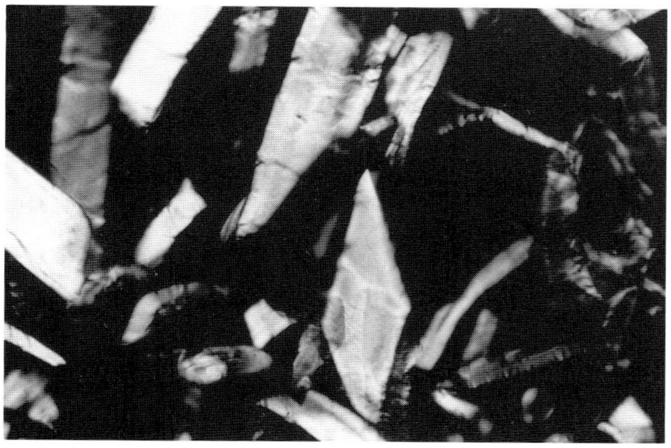

Fig. 4.59. Paper towel, polarized view. Cellulose is strongly birefringent.

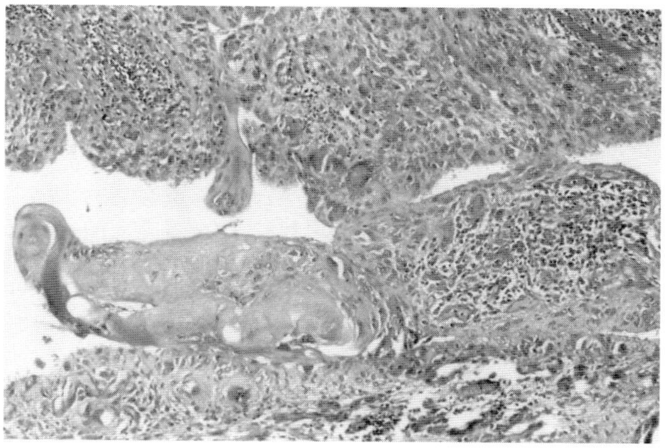

Fig. 4.60. Low-power view of synovial hyperplasia with chronic inflammation in artificial joint implant.

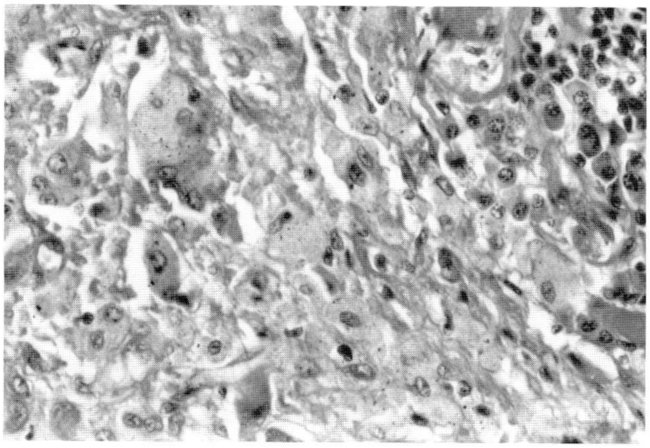

Fig. 4.61. Higher power view of histiocytes with fine black granules, which are from metallic wear debris of an artificial joint.

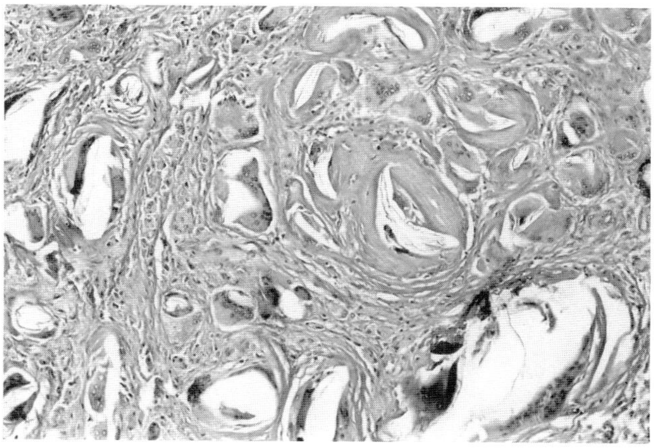

Fig. 4.62. Methyl methacrylate and polyethylene in knee replacement. Note prominent foreign body giant cell with clear spaces, which were occupied by methyl methacrylate. Normal processing dissolves methyl methacrylate. Polyethylene is retained after processing and appears as highly refractile, clear fragments in giant cells.

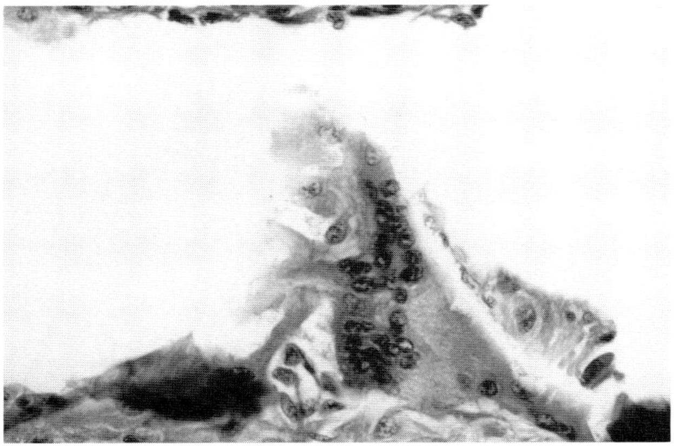

Fig. 4.63. Methyl methacrylate, in artificial joint. There is a large angulated space with foreign body giant cell reaction.

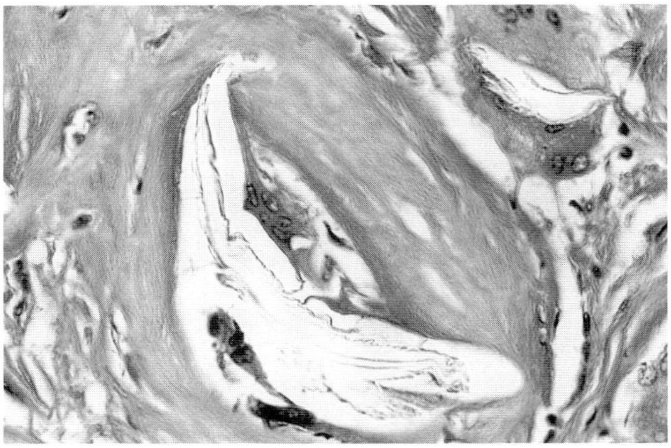

Fig. 4.64. Polyethylene, in artificial joint. There is refractile material with a foreign body reaction.

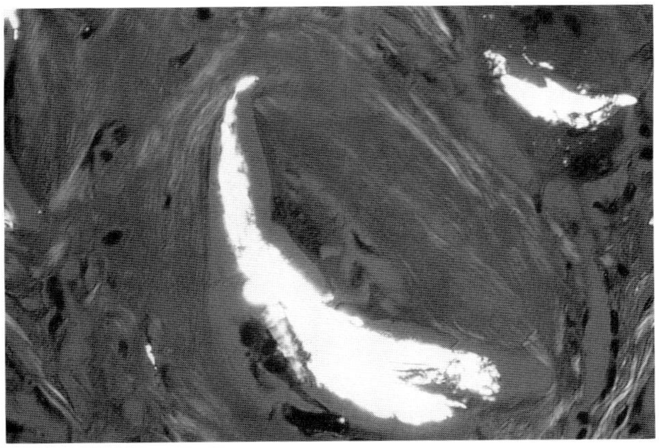

Fig. 4.65. Polarized view of polyethylene. The material is highly anisotropic.

5

Organic Materials

Pathologic examination of tissue may include plant or animal food material in the gastrointestinal (GI) tract, extending from the oral cavity to the rectum. Retained food is commonly seen in diverticuli, as well as in other nonmoving segments. Food material may be present within the abdominal or thoracic cavities due to trauma, infection, rupture of a viscus, or tumor. Plant materials seen outside the GI tract in tissues are most often due to aspiration or subcutaneous implantation. The cellular response to plant and animal matter is a typical foreign body reaction, composed of histiocytes, lymphocytes, and giant cells, sometimes forming granulomas. Fragments of the material may be seen within giant cells. Ordinarily, a diagnosis of plant or foreign material is rendered, without further specification. A description of common plant and animal food materials follows to allow for more definite identification.

Aspirated material may be either plant or animal in origin and often is a mixture of both plant and animal origin. Plant and animal materials are distinguished by features of **plant** cells which are not seen in animal cells: cell walls, plastids, and starch grains. Cell walls are the most distinctive feature. They are poorly stained by hematoxylin–eosin (H&E) and appear as refractile, stacked geometric shapes. Polarization light microscopy brings out cell walls. Histochemical staining for cellulose, the cell walls' main component, may also highlight the presence of cell walls. Plastids are intracytoplasmic structures with limiting membranes and function as manufacturing and storage areas for pigment, fats, proteins, or starches. Grains contain starch and can be easily identified because of the massive quantities in which they occur. Another distinguishing feature of plant cells includes their sometimes remarkably large size and the range of colors that can be present. In general, differentiation of various plant types may be made on the basis of examining the number of starch grains, the cell size, and cell wall thickness (Table 5.1) Histochemical stains may be used to recognize various plant components. For example, inulin or arabic gum may be identified using Szederkenyi and Jozsa stains. Starch is strongly stained by periodic acid–Schiff (PAS). Cellulose is demonstrated by selective cotton dyes, with and without cellulase digestion. The Maacz stain identifies lignin.

Pollen grains are present in the air, with high numbers of grains at predictable times, depending upon the climate. Pollen may be found in a variety of tissue locations, including the respiratory tract, gastrointestinal tract, and urine. Its appearance in tissues mirrors the seasonal increases. Pollen grains

Table 5.1 Differentiation of Plant Types

	Starch Grains	Cell Size	Cell Wall Thickness
Legumes	+++	++	+
Grains	++++	+/−	+
Leafy	−	++++	++
Fruit	+	+++	+
Nuts	+++	++	+
Roots	++++	++	+
Wood	−	++	++++

(+ = present, slight degree; ++++ = present, marked; − = absent)

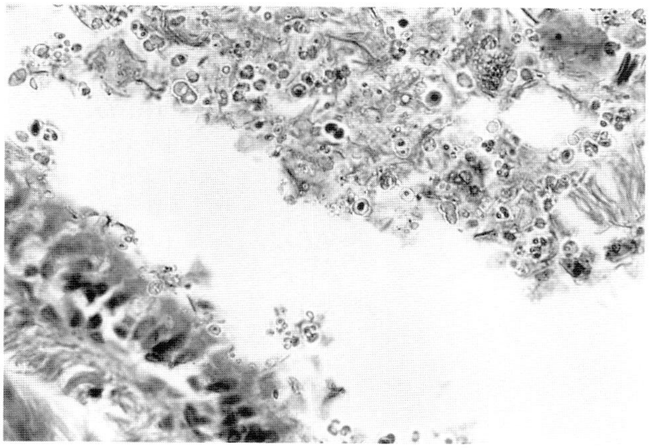

Fig. 5.1. Aspirated food in bronchus (processed starch material). Numerous refractile round starch granules are evident within the lumen of the bronchus.

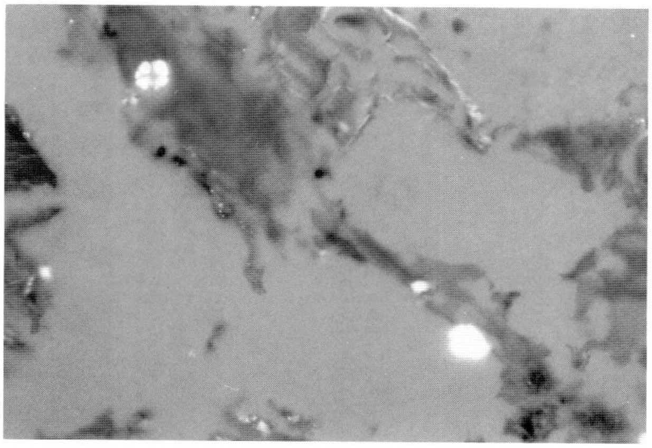

Fig. 5.2. Starch granules with polarized light. The characteristic "Maltese cross" configuration is seen in the upper left corner.

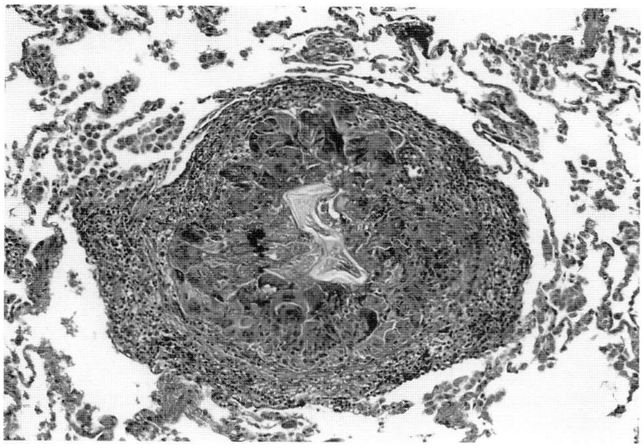

Fig. 5.3. Aspiration of carrots, with formation of granuloma. Cellulose of plant cell walls is recognized as clear, linear material forming polygonal spaces.

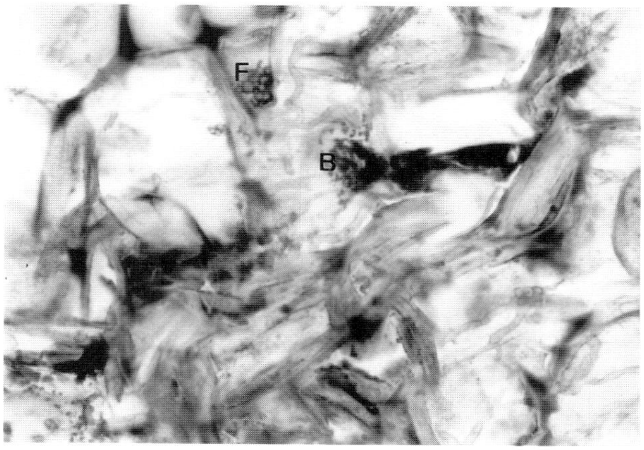

Fig. 5.4. Plant material obstructing small bowel. Retained cell walls with polygonal matrix showing collapse. Bacteria (B) and fungi (F) are growing within.

are highly variable in size and shape, depending upon the plant of origin; however, common characteristics include lack of nucleus and refractile cell wall. Ziehl-Neelsen (carbol fuchsin) will demonstrate pollen grains.

Legumes are edible seeds, including lentils, peas, and beans. The relatively dense nature of these vegetables and their oval shape make aspiration a real possibility. The general appearance of a legume is an outer shell composed of linear arrays of columnar cells with yellow-brown granules, with an inner mass of cells containing starch grains. These grains appear as glassy, ovoid, light blue intracytoplasmic globules on H&E stain and are strongly PAS-positive. Polarization of these globules shows their "Maltese cross" configuration. These grains are separated by a densely eosinophilic cytoplasm.

Other edible seeds are known as **nuts**, such as walnuts, almonds, cashews. Nuts are high in oil content and are characterized by an internal matrix of cells with densely eosinophilic granules of variable sizes. Like legumes, the size, shape, and density of nuts may lead to aspiration and subsequently respiratory compromise.

Starchy vegetables include the potato, a root vegetable. Microscopically, the potato contains a pigmented outer surface (periderm), a cortex of small starch-rich cells, a zone of conducting cells, and a central portion of large starch-rich cells. After cooking, the cell walls are partially disrupted. If the potato has been fried, the cellular response may include numerous foamy histiocytes because of the increased oil content.

Grains are small hard seeds and include corn, rice, wheat, barley, and oat. The external portions are proteinaceous aleurone and the husk. The inner grains consist of an oily embryo (germ) and a starchy endosperm. Cooked, processed grains appear as amorphous eosinophilic material, with characteristics similar to caseous necrosis. Corn contains central amorphous eosinophilic material and irregular basophilic deposits and a surrounding honeycomb-like matrix of cell walls.

Commonly aspirated fruit include the "stone" or drupe **fruits**, which can be defined as a fleshy fruit having a hard central stone containing a seed. Examples of the drupe fruits include peaches, apricots, plums, and cherries. The stones may be aspirated, but are not commonly sectioned, because of their hard consistency. The fleshy fruits are characterized by an external skin layer of small, oval cells containing pigment. Pigment is compartmentalized in discrete intracytoplasmic structures, the plastids. The inner portions of fruits are composed of a matrix of oval cell walls, without distinct nuclei. This inner matrix contains watery, faintly eosinophilic fluid, which may be lightly stained by PAS. Other fruits include the berries (grape, blueberry, and persimmon), aggregate fruits (strawberry and raspberry), and pomes (apples and pears).

Botanically, herbaceous annual plants bear fruits, some of which are popularly recognized as **vegetables**, including the tomato, eggplants, squash, and okra. Others, such as melons, are regarded as fruits, depending on the sugar content of the pulp. The tomato contains massive amount of water, causing the cells to balloon up into extreme sizes. Leafy vegetables such as lettuce contain predominantly water. The residual matrix is a honeycomb arrangement of cell walls and veins (xylem and phloem) which act to carry water and nutrients. The smallest branches of veins appear as coiled tubes (tracheids), seemingly randomly distributed in the leaves. Veins are present throughout

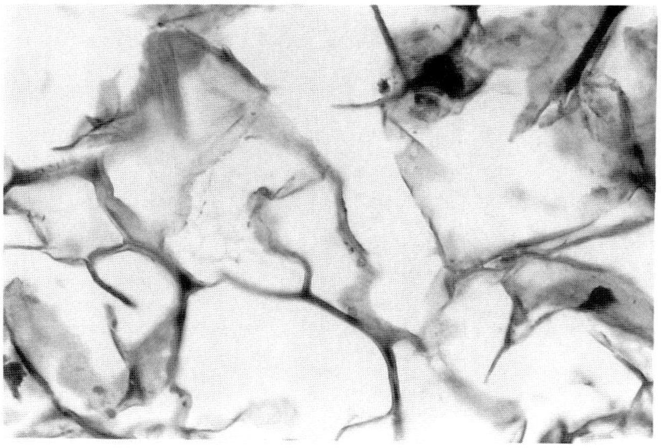

Fig. 5.5. Plant material obstructing small bowel. Note the matrix of cell walls. Intracellular contents and nuclei are not apparent.

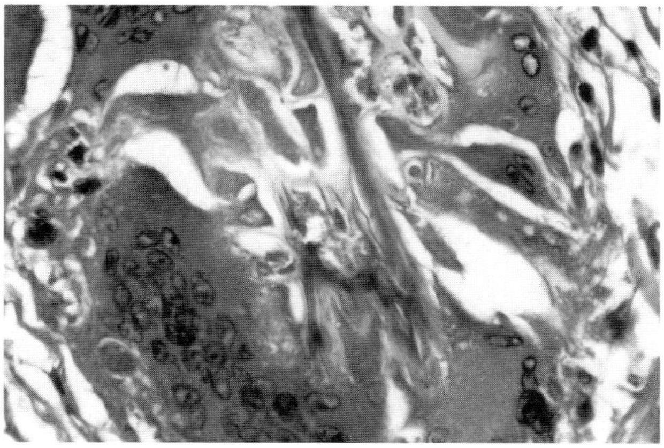

Fig. 5.6. Vegetable material in hernia sac. There is a foreign body giant cell reaction. Cellulose cell walls are retained.

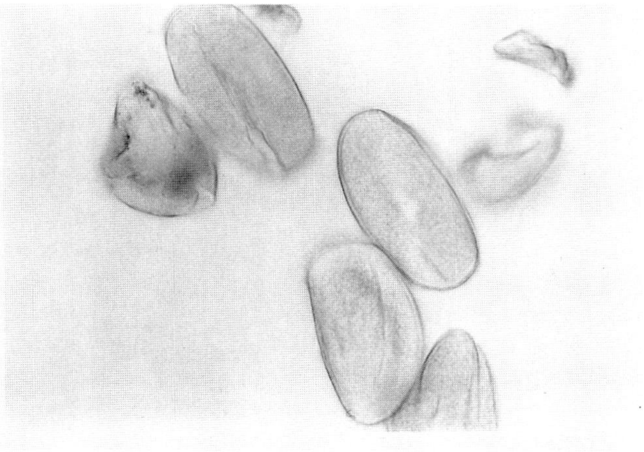

Fig. 5.7. Pollen grains, rose. Note the thick, refractile cell walls. Internal structures are not seen.

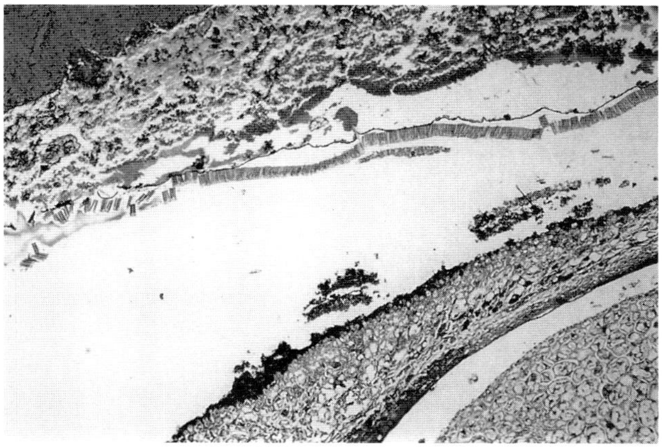

Fig. 5.8. Kidney bean in necrotic colon. The external layer is composed of cellulose material, in closely packed linear bands, perpendicular to the internal contents.

plants but may appear more prominantly in leaves. The leaves quickly wilt with body heat because of the high water content, and they rarely cause an aspiration death.

Technically a plant, mushrooms are an edible fungus. Microscopically, both branching hyphae and yeast forms may be seen. The specific type of mushroom dictates the width of hyphae, branching characteristics, and yeast shapes. Silver and PAS stains demonstrate the fungal nature of mushrooms well, if necessary.

Nonhuman **animal** material found in humans is typically food that has either been aspirated or is present in the gastrointestinal tract. Most meat is pure muscle tissue, similar to human skeletal muscle. It may sometimes be grossly recognized, if aspiration of a large piece causes death. Microscopically, muscle from common domestic animals appears similar. Meat is composed of eosinophilic fibers, with peripheral nuclei. Cross striations may be present, but may be partially lost after prolonged cooking. Fluid is commonly present between fibers. Adipose tissue content is variable, with beef often containing large amounts.

Processed meat has a more varied appearance. Hot dogs or sausages may be aspirated, causing death because of lack of aeration beyond the dense tissue which lodges in the trachea or other airway space. Microscopically, processed meat contains some skeletal muscle, but other mesenchymal tissues are admixed, such as fibrous, adipose, cartilage, as well as air holes and other fillers, including vegetable fragments.

Other organs may also be consumed, most frequently liver. Although liver is softer in consistency than most meat, it may still cause suffocation. Chicken liver may sometimes be recognized by its nucleated red blood cells.

Rarely, massive trauma may cause **embolization** of fragments of human tissues, including bone marrow and liver, to other sites, typically lung.

Organic materials that act as foreign bodies in **subcutaneous tissue** include hairs, which incite a chronic inflammatory and giant cell response. Hairs are composed of three layers: the cuticle (scale), cortex, and medulla. The cuticle consists of overlapping cells on the surface. The cortex is composed primarily of keratin and forms the structural support of the hair. Pigment is usually present. Medulla is the central portion and is variably present on a cross section of hair. Color and size, as well as other cuticle, cortical, and medullary characteristics have been used to determine the origin of hair in forensic applications. A common surgical specimen is the pilonidal cyst, which is essentially a sinus tract composed of implanted hair and the resultant foreign body reaction.

Insects may embed themselves into the skin and subcutaneous tissues, such as *Demodex follicularum, Dermatobia hominis* (human botfly), *Cordylobia anthropophaga* (tumbu fly), and *Cochliomyis hominivorax* (primary screwworm). Insects may be identified by their thick polysaccharide coat, the chitin. Chitin appears as an eosinophilic semitransparent layer surrounding the organism. Internal organs can be identified. Nematodes also are surrounded by eosinophilic cuticles and can be found in the subcutaneous tissues, as well as other organs. The human host reaction is variable, but often includes eosinophils, chronic inflammatory cells, and foreign body giant cells.

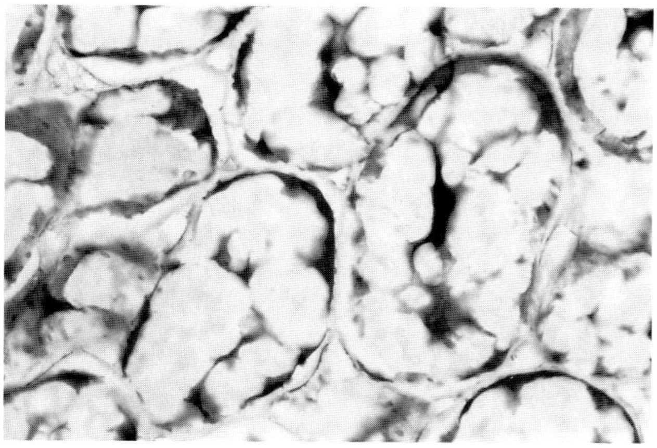

Fig. 5.9. Higher power of central cells of kidney bean. Cells store starch within cytoplasmic granules, which appear in typical "Maltese cross" configuration upon polarization microscopy. Nuclei are dark and centrally located.

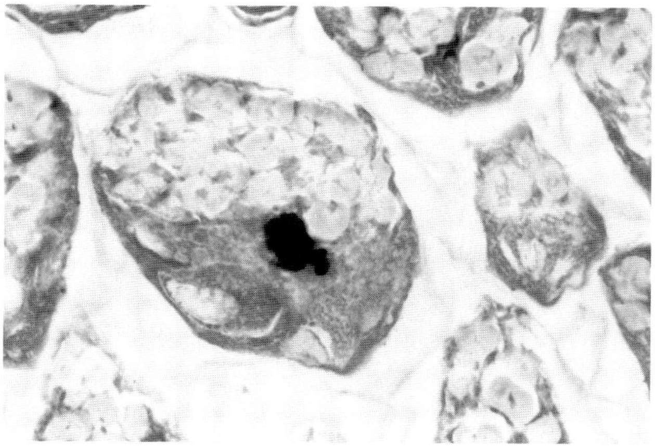

Fig. 5.10. Pea, starch-containing cell. The numerous starch granules are light blue on H&E stain. The cells appear overstuffed, and nuclei are not well visualized. There is an evident space between the cell and cell wall.

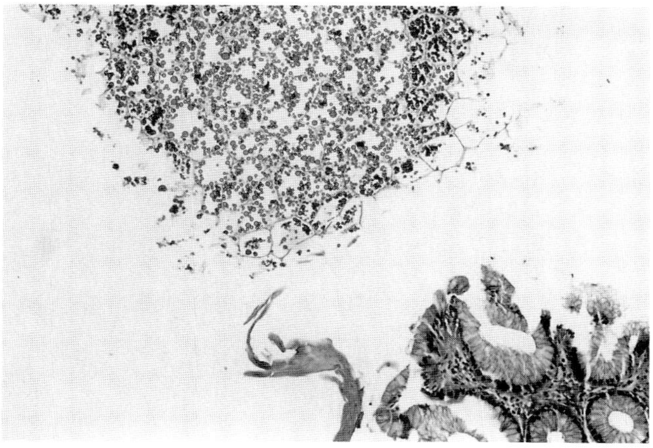

Fig. 5.11. Esophageal–gastric junction, with fragment of nut in lumen. Note the matrix of cell walls, with numerous eosinophilic intracytoplasmic globules, which are characteristic of nuts.

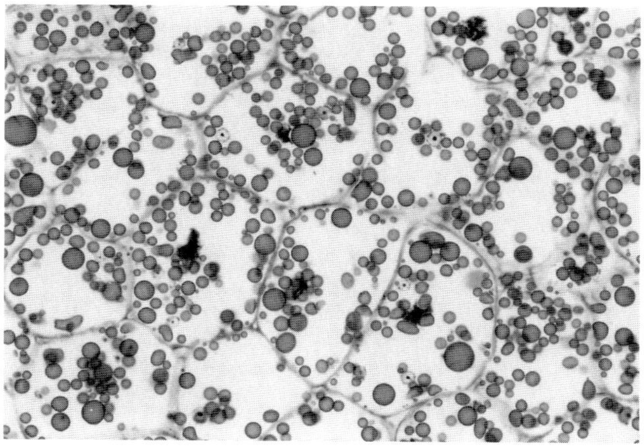

Fig. 5.12. Peanut. The cells are in a polygonal matrix, with numerous intracytoplasmic hyaline globules of different sizes.

Plant foreign materials in subcutaneous tissue include wood fragments, thorns, or spines. These materials may be embedded during the course of percutaneous trauma from household furniture, building parts, yard, park, etc.

Wood fragments contain a large amount of cellulose and have extremely dense cell walls. The cell walls are usually empty and may be lined with tannins, gums, dyes, or crystals. The main conduction system of the tree can be present as longitudinal vessels or horizontal rays. Bark is the living, growing portion of the tree trunk and is composed of several layers, the epidermis, cortex, pericycle, and phloem. The cells of the bark are typically smaller than those from the central portion of the tree trunk. Typically bark is pigmented, with numerous yellow brown granules.

Thorns or spines are modified leaves which end in a spike. For example, an embedded cactus spike elicits a giant cell response. Careful examination may reveal that the giant cells contain sharply spiculated particles which are PAS-positive; spikes may also be present free in dermis.

Finally, foods may also contain other foreign material, which cause injury to the perioral region or the gastrointestinal tract. Common objects in this category include glass, metal, or plastic shards. Descriptions of these materials are presented in other Chapters.

BIBLIOGRAPHY

Boon AP: Histomorphometry and immunohistochemistry of beef sausages. *J Clin Pathol* 43:435, 1990.

Covell JL, Feldman PS: Fine needle aspiration pneumonia. *Acta Cytol* 28:77–80, 1984.

Jozsa L, Reffy A, Demel S: Histochemical and histophysical detection and specification of foreign bodies in human tissues. *Zentralbl.allg.Pathol.pathol.Anat* 135:675–684, 1989.

Kaplan SL, Gnepp DR, Katzenstein AA, et al: Miliary pulmonary nodules due to aspirated vegetable particles. *J Ped* 92:448–450, 1978.

Lovas GL, Howell RE, Peters E, et al: Starch artifacts in oral cytologic specimens. *Oral Surg Oral Med Oral Pathol* 60:195–196, 1985.

Watson RE, Stewart C: Experimental oral foreign body reactions: vegetable materials. *Oral Surg Oral Med Oral Pathol* 71:312–316, 1991.

Weaver KM, Novak PM, Naylor B: Vegetable cell contaminants in cytologic specimens. *Acta Cytol* 25:210–214, 1981.

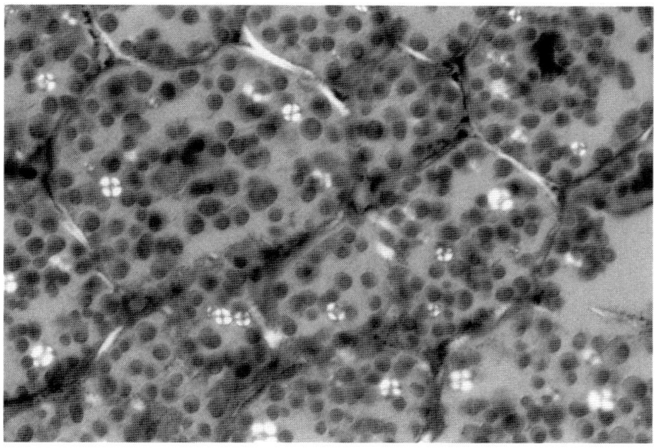

Fig. 5.13. Peanut, polarized light microscopy. Polarization brings out the starch granules within the cytoplasm.

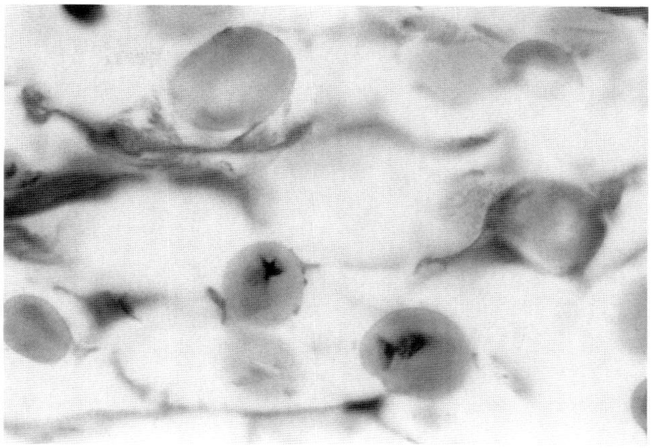

Fig. 5.14. Potato, a starchy root vegetable. Cells of the potato may reach quite large sizes and are filled with fluid and giant starch grains.

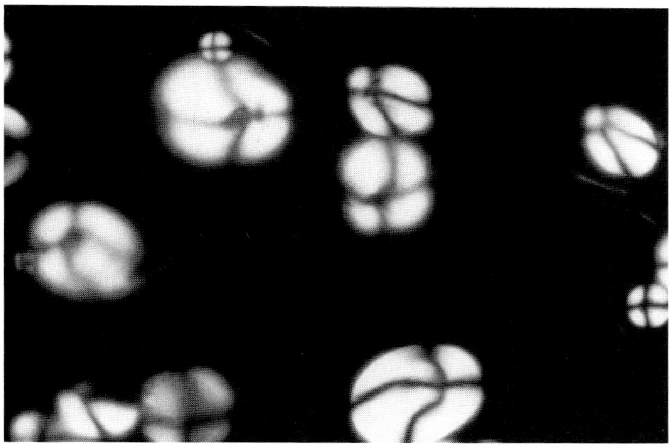

Fig. 5.15. Potato, polarized light microscopy. The starch grains of the potato are similar to the configuration of other starchy vegetables but are larger in size than most.

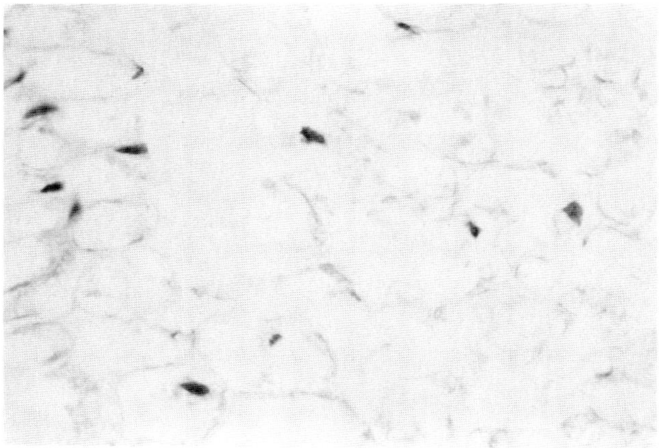

Fig. 5.16. Corn, outer matrix. The outer portion of a corn kernel contains an epidermal layer and fluid-containing cells within a matrix of cell walls.

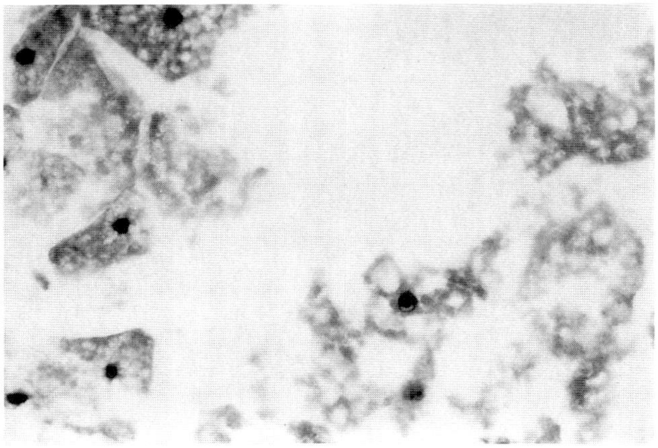

Fig. 5.17. Corn, central portion of kernel. The central cells in a kernel of corn have round, dark nuclei and contain numerous starch granules.

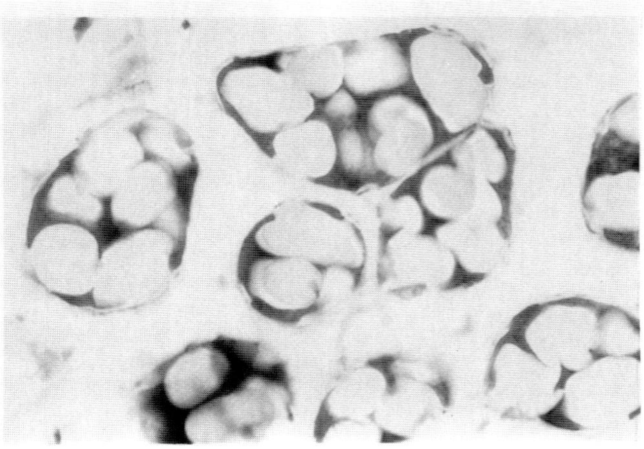

Fig. 5.18. Rice, cooked. A few cells are still intact, overstuffed with pale blue globules (starch grains). Nuclei are dark and distorted by the starch globules.

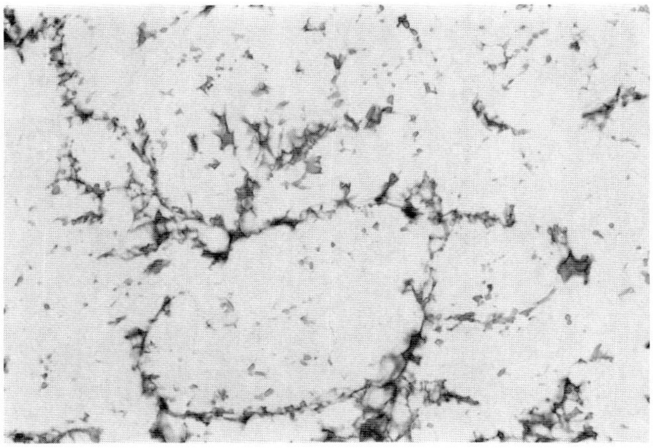

Fig. 5.19. Rice, cooked. This rice was in excess water, and the cell walls have ruptured. There is a sea of amorphous starch material, including fragments of starch granules and the bare outlines of cell walls.

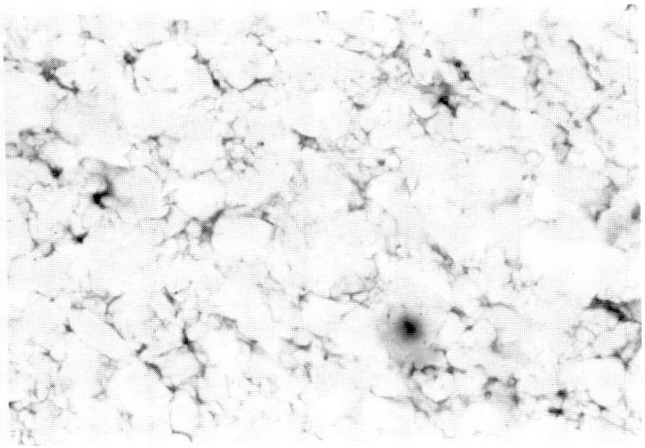

Fig. 5.20. Pasta. Microscopically, cooked pasta consists of an amorphous matrix, with partial preservation of cells walls and "Maltese cross" starch grains.

Fig. 5.21. Tomato. The cells of a tomato contain large amounts of fluid. Cell walls are pushed far apart, so that the field contains mostly liquid. They are variable in size and can reach extreme magnitudes.

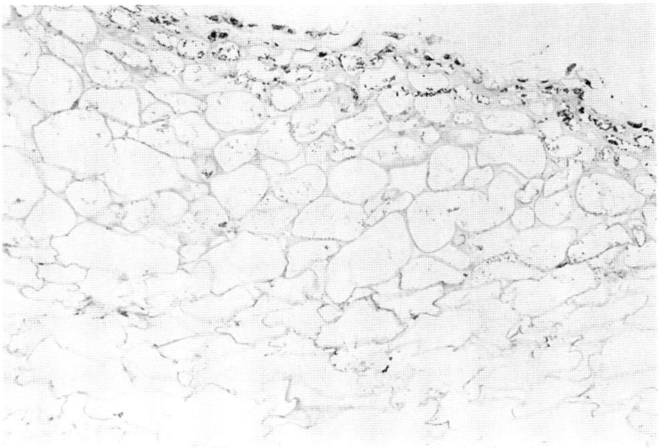

Fig. 5.22. Apple. The cells of an apple are filled primarily with fluid. Note the epidermis of the apple at the top, with relatively small, pigment-containing cells.

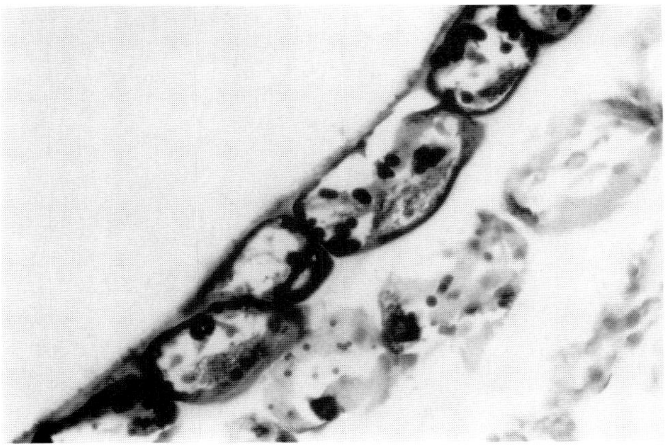

Fig. 5.23. Blueberry, epidermis. Darkly pigmented plastids are easily visualized in the outer layer of the blueberry.

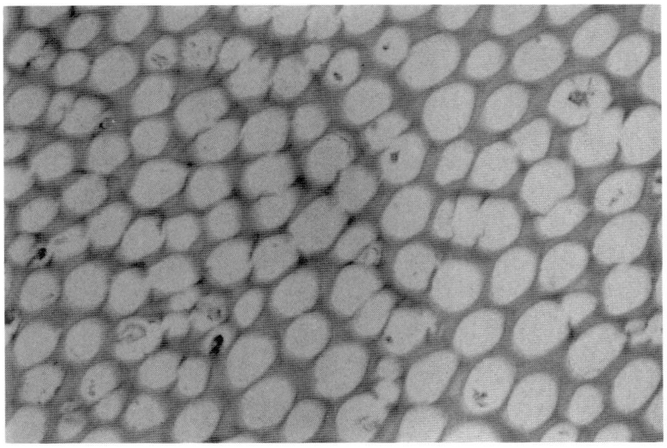

Fig. 5.24. Celery, fibrous area. Note the uniform thick cell walls.

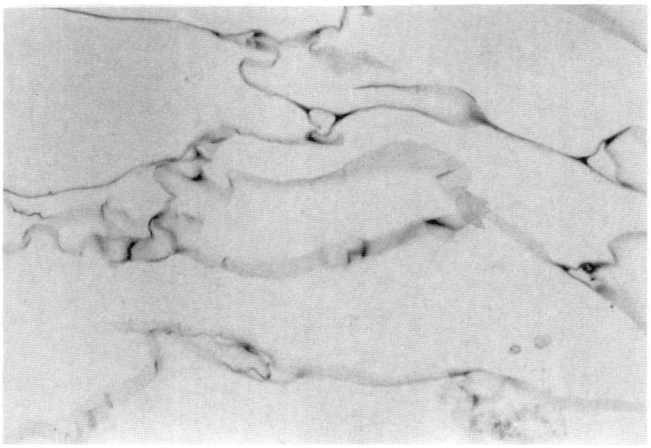

Fig. 5.25. Celery, body. These cells contain abundant fluid and are larger than the fibrous area cells, with thinner cell walls.

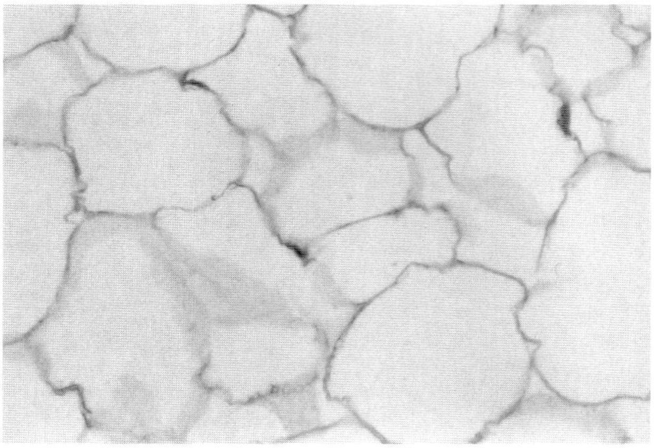

Fig. 5.26. Cabbage. The matrix of cell walls is relatively uniform in cabbage leaves. The cells are filled with fluid.

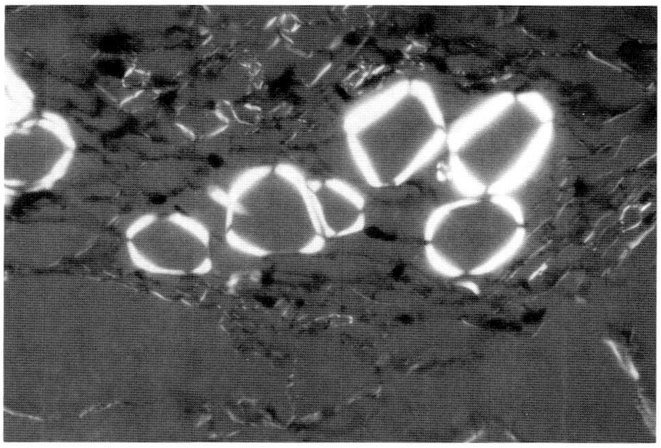

Fig. 5.27. Carrot, polarized light microscopy. Veins are in cross section. The polarized view shows marked birefringence of veins in comparison to other plant cells.

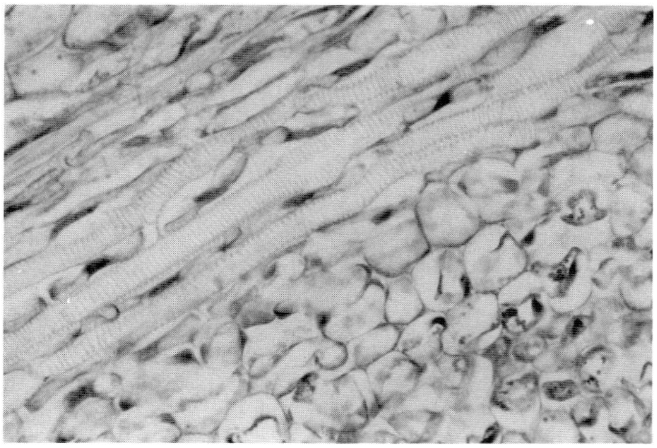

Fig. 5.28. Bean sprout with longitudinal view of veins, in between starch-containing cells. The veins appear as stretched out spirals.

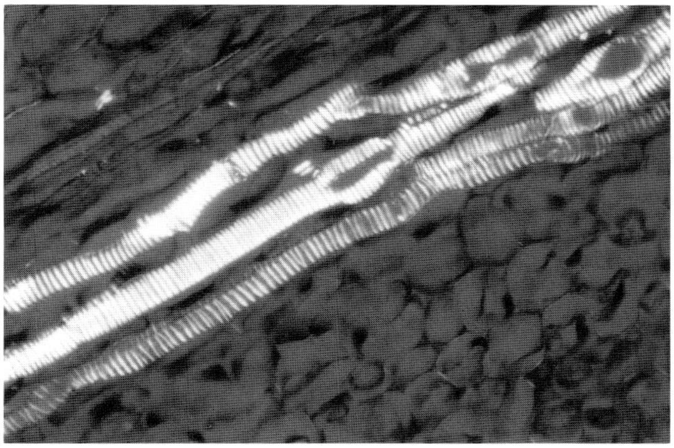

Fig. 5.29. Bean sprout, polarized view. The bright birefringence of the veins is evident.

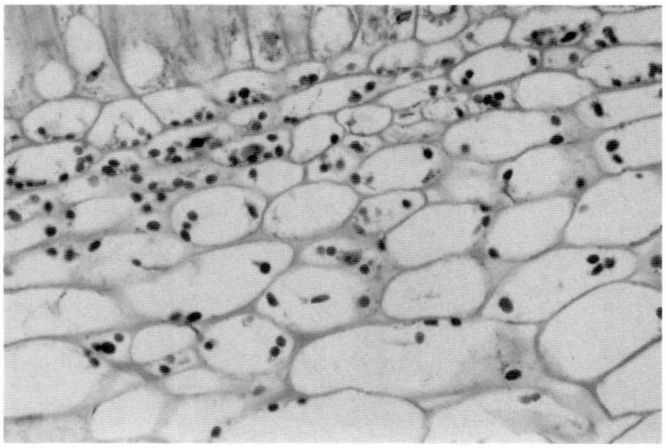

Fig. 5.30. Cucumber, skin at top. Ovoid cells with large amount of water. Ovoid intracytoplasmic plastids.

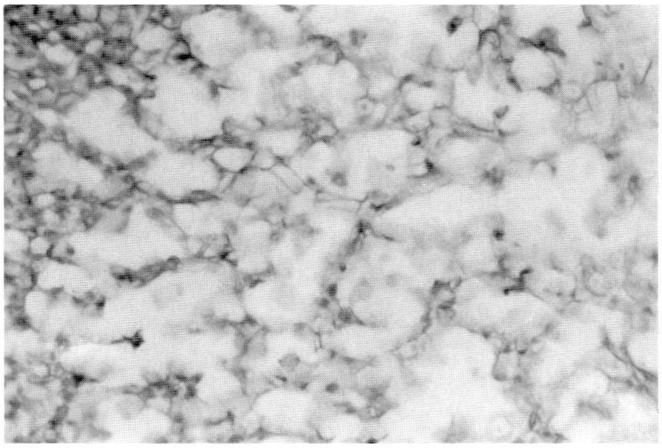

Fig. 5.31. Mushroom. Fungal hyphe make up the bulk of mushrooms, typically seen in anatomosing strands.

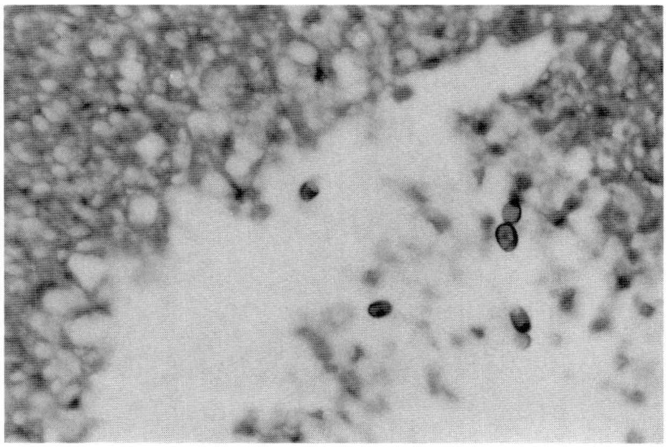

Fig. 5.32. Mushroom. A few budding yeasts are present, with hyphae in the background, in a different plane of focus.

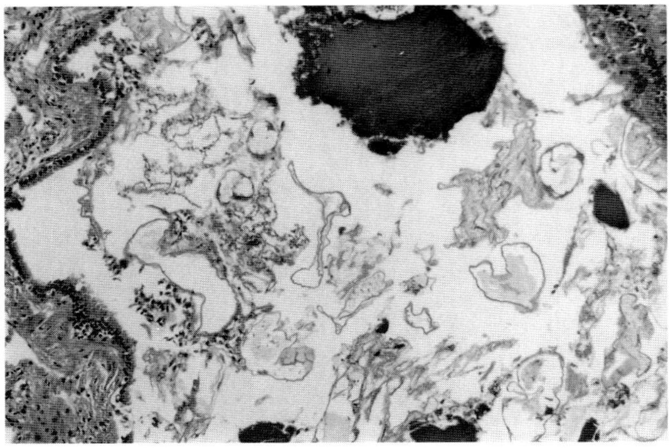

Fig. 5.33. Lung with aspirated food material. Photograph shows a dilated bronchiole with starch cells from bean, muscle fibers, as well as other miscellaneous fibers.

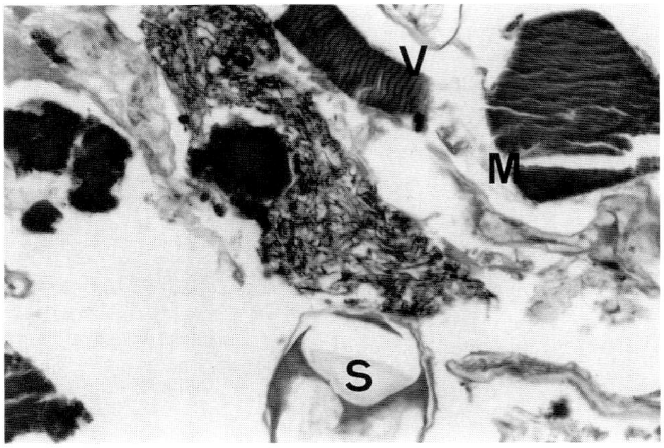

Fig. 5.34. Lung, aspirated food material, high power. The structure of the mixed food materials is evident here: starch cell (S), muscle fiber (M), and plant vessel (V).

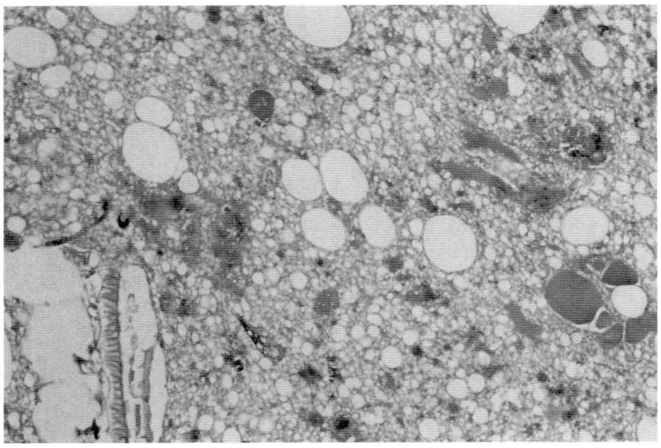

Fig. 5.35. Hot dog. Note numerous large empty vacuoles with mesenchymal cellular fragments (muscle, cartilege, bone, fibrous tissue, vessels), as well as a few vegetable fibers.

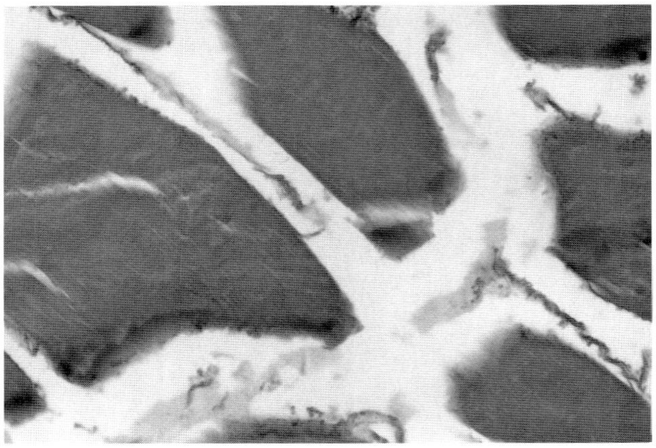

Fig. 5.36. Tunafish (canned). Spaced muscle fibers with poorly visualized nuclei.

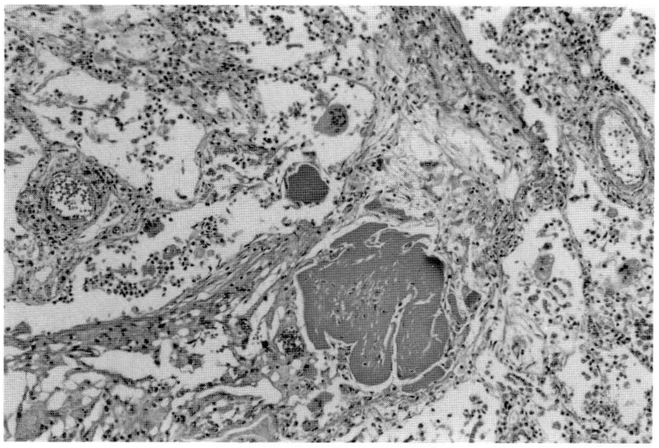

Fig. 5.37. Lung, with aspirated cooked meat. Note dense eosinophilic muscle fibers with peripheral nuclei. After cooking, cross striations are less prominent.

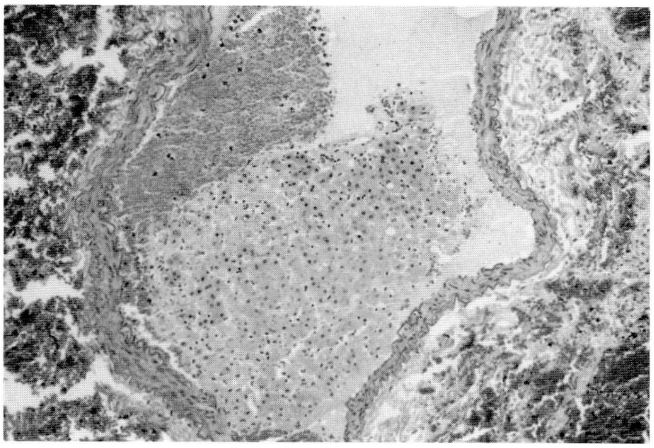

Fig. 5.38. Liver embolus in pulmonary artery. Massive abdominal trauma resulted in embolization of liver. The tissue fragment is recognizable as essentially normal human liver.

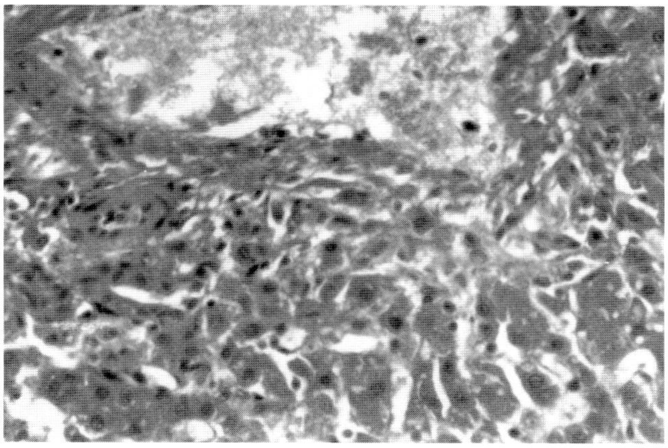

Fig. 5.39. Chicken liver in glottis, found in a choking victim. The chicken liver has been cooked and thus nuclear and cytoplasmic details are fuzzy.

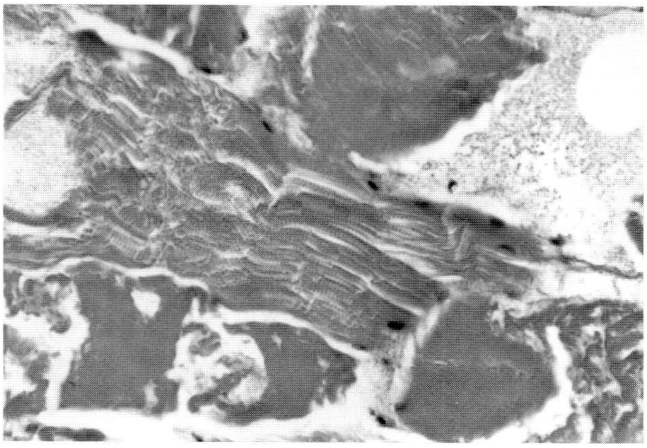

Fig. 5.40. Swordfish (cooked). Cross striations are present in cytoplasm and nuclei are peripheral. Fluid surrounds some of the fibers.

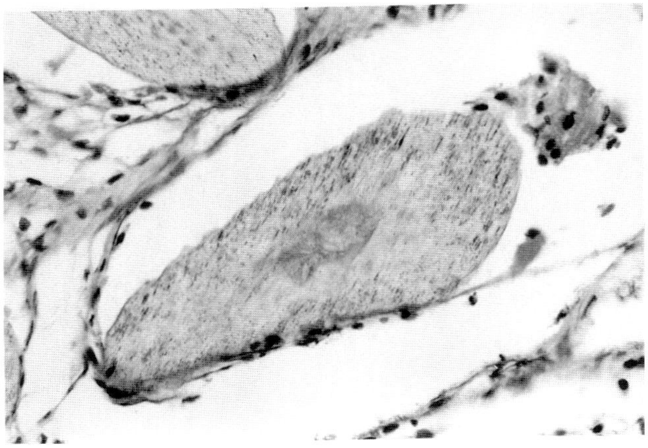

Fig. 5.41. Hair, pilonidal cyst. The pilonidal cyst is a sinus tract composed of implanted hair. The oval cross sections of hair have pigment in the cortical layers and a medulla is present centrally.

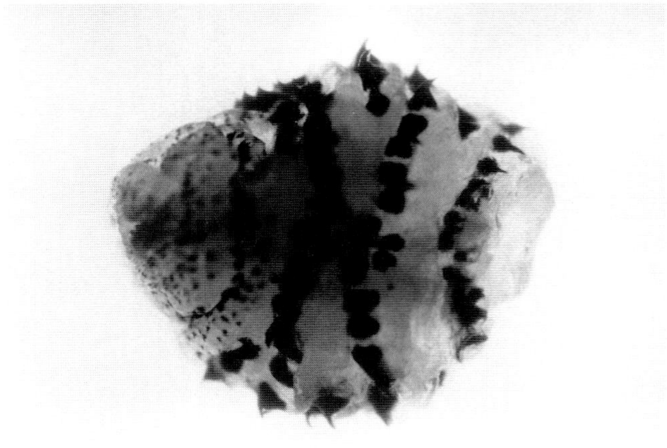

Fig. 5.42. Human botfly (*Dermatobia hominis*). This insect was removed from the subcutaneous tissue of a patient who had recently traveled to Central America. Note the thick translucent chitin layer.

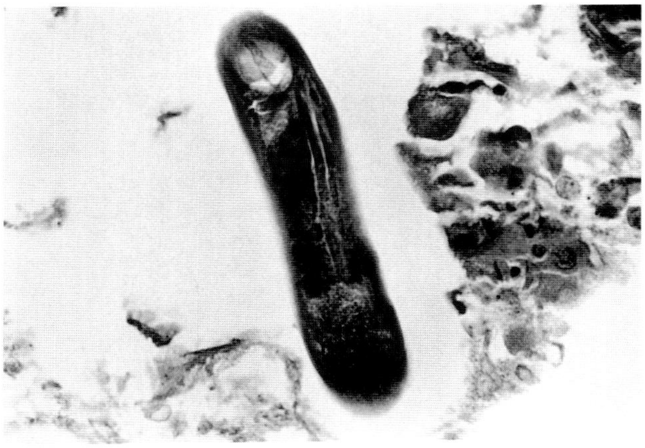

Fig. 5.43. Strongyloides. Strongyloides stercoalis usually infests the intestine, but may have skin dissemination in immunocompromised hosts. The elongated form with a thick external layer is characteristic, as are the internal gut contents.

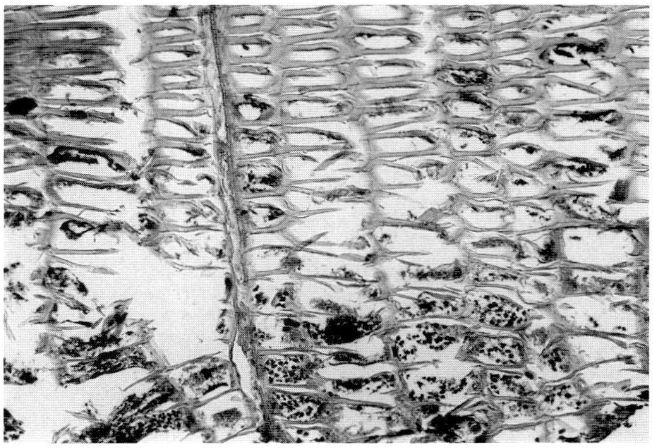

Fig. 5.44. Wood splinter removed from subcutaneous tissue. Wood is composed of a regular polygonal arrangement of cell walls.

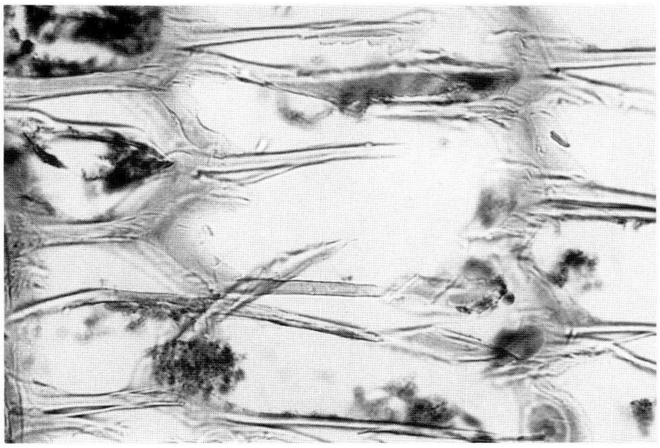

Fig. 5.45. Wood splinter, high power. Note the extremely thick cellulose cell wall matrix and essentially empty cell space.

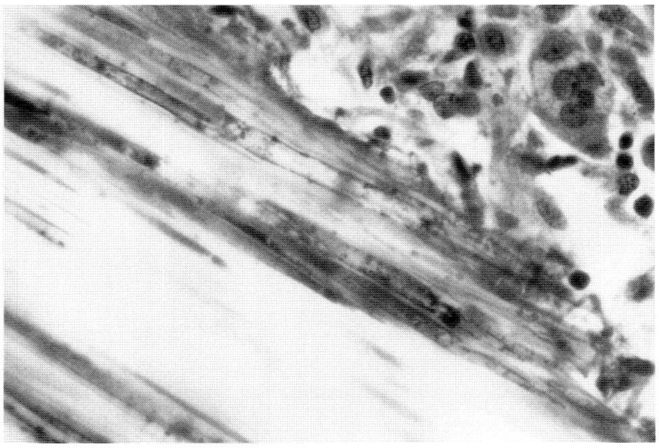

Fig. 5.46. Wood splinter, after 15 months. Dense refractile linear material with chronic inflammatory response. In this case, the polygonal shapes of the cell walls are not well visualized.

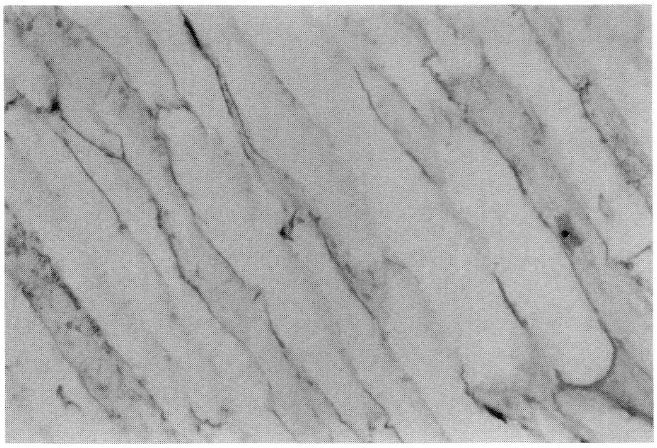

Fig. 5.47. Thorn. The thorn has characteristics of both stem and wood, with thick cell walls and poorly visualized cells.

6 Pigments

Pigments occur widely in tissue. The colors seen in tissue sections span the visible spectrum, from the primary colors of red (blood), yellow (bile), and blue (iron) to brown and black, which are mixtures of all colors. Most of the pigment seen in the surgical pathology laboratory is naturally occurring, or **endogenous.** Endogenous pigments may be normal (skin pigmentation), due to aging (lipofuscin) or pathologic (accumulation of excess iron or copper). Other pigments are from **exogenous** sources, due to the patients' choice (tattoos), inhalation (carbon), surgery (inks), or laboratory processing (inks).

ENDOGENOUS PIGMENTS

Melanin is probably the best known pigment, as it is the source of skin pigmentation. Other sites for natural deposits of melanin include the mucosa, particularly in heavily pigmented individuals, as well as the eye and other neural crest–derived tissues. Melanin pigment may be increased with drug therapy or after injury, such as in postinflammatory pigmentation of the skin. Post-therapeutic pigmentation with melanin may result on light exposed skin after tranquilizers, minocycline, amiodarone, and cardiac drugs. Melanosis has also been described in mucosal sites, such as in the cervix after cryotherapy for squamous dysplasia. Microscopically, melanin appears as fine brown or black granules in melanocytes or melanophages. The distinction of melanin from other pigments is crucial when making the diagnosis of a malignant melanoma. Special stains that demonstrate melanin are based on the silver staining of the granules and include Grimelius, Masson-Fontana, Sevier-Monger, and Warthin-Starry. These stains are not completely specific for melanin, and the interpretation of positive staining should be coupled with appropriate histology and pattern of staining; that is, of fine intracytoplasmic granules in cells that sometimes have a dendritic pattern. Melanin can be bleached by potassium permanganate, which may allow better visualization of nuclear characteristics in a heavily pigmented tumor. Potassium permanganate has been used to differentiate melanin from other pigments, but the technique is not specific enough to be reliable. Melanosomes, the specific cellular organelle for melanin, can be identified by electron microscopy. Immunopathologic stains (S100, HMB45) are useful in the distinction of melanoma from other malignant neoplasms, but do not specifically stain melanin granules.

Hemosiderin is a complex of iron and protein (ferritin), which represents the cellular form of stored iron. Microscopically, hemosiderin appears as coarse golden-brown granules within cells. If one turns down the condenser light, the granules take on an "apple green" color. Hemosiderin may be present in virtually any tissue and is seen as a product of red blood cell breakdown in the marrow, spleen, or liver, or may occur as a result of hemorrhage. Special stains to identify hemosiderin include various iron stains. Perls' Prussian blue stains ferric iron a blue color; almost all tissue iron is in ferric state. Turnbull blue reaction stains ferrous salts blue. Quincke's and Tirmann-Schmeltzer reactions stain both ferrous and ferric iron. Quincke's reaction stains iron green-brown or black, whereas Tirmann-Schmeltzer reaction stains iron dark blue.

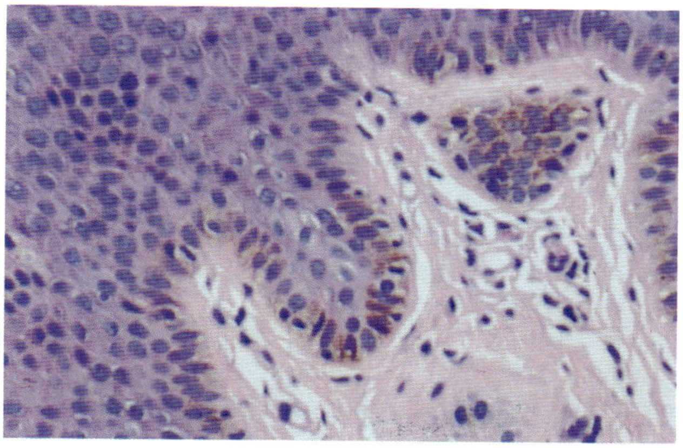

Fig. 6.1. Melanin pigment, skin. Melanocytes are normally present in all individuals, with darker skinned persons having a heavier deposition of melanin. The pigment appears as fine brown intracellular granules.

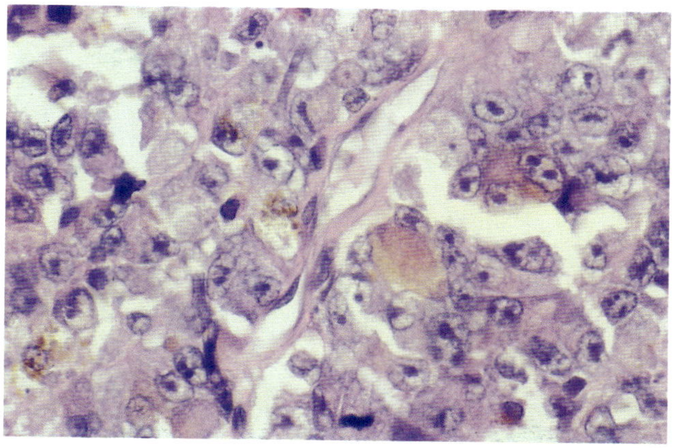

Fig. 6.2. Melanin pigment, melanoma of skin. Melanoma is a malignant tumor of melanocytes, and many of the malignant cells will contain the dusty brown melanin pigment. However, hemosiderin may also be present in histiocytes in the same vicinity. Hemosiderin is distinguished from melanin by having larger, coarser granules, and a green refractility when the condenser is turned down.

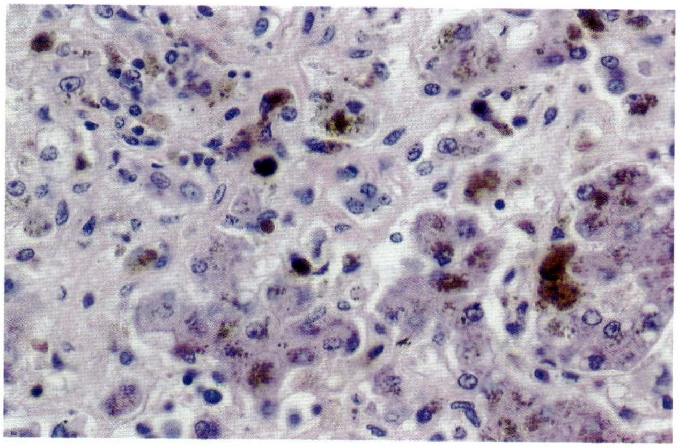

Fig. 6.3. Liver, hemosiderin. There are numerous iron granules within hepatocytes in this patient with primary hemochromatosis.

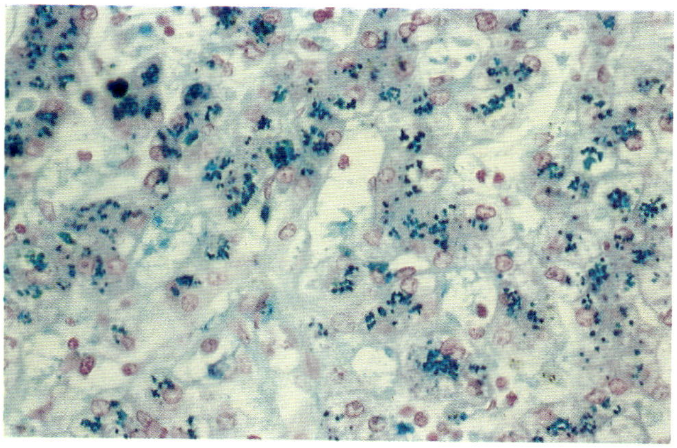

Fig. 6.4. Liver, hemosiderin, Prussian blue stain. The Prussian blue stain is markedly positive in the hemosiderin granules in the above patient.

Dark pigmentation of the mucosal surface of the colon is found in **melanosis coli.** This condition is associated with ingestion of anthracene-derived bowel cathartics. Microscopically, macrophages containing a lipofuscin-like, brown to black pigment are present in the lamina propria and even the muscularis propria of the colon. Prolonged usage of anthracene laxatives may lead to pigmented histiocytes in the draining mesenteric lymph nodes. Silver stains are positive and the pigment can be bleached by peroxide. The muscularis propria may be atrophic, and neuronal abnormalities of the myenteric plexus can be demonstrated by silver stains.

Hematin (hemozoin, malarial pigment, schistosomal pigment) appears as brown to black granules inside macrophages. It is seen in the liver and spleen with malaria and schistosomal infections or severe hemolytic anemia. In malaria, the trophozoite forms this complex from the breakdown of red blood cells. Similarly, in schistosomiasis, the pigment is due to regurgitation of blood breakdown products from the schistosome organism. It is moderately birefringent on polarized light and does not stain for iron. **Formalin pigment** is an artifact of tissue fixation in acid formalin, and consists of acid hematin (see Chapter 1). It is particularly prominent in tissues containing large amounts of blood, such as the spleen. It has the same characteristics as the malarial pigment described above; however, formalin pigment typically appears as a precipitant within tissue, often located in a different plane of focus, and is not seen in association with a macrophage tissue response.

Bile pigments include biliverdin, conjugated or unconjugated bilirubin, or mixtures of these compounds. In the breakdown of red blood cells, hemoglobin is separated into heme and globin. The iron is removed from heme to form biliverdin, which appears as a green pigment. Biliverdin is further decomposed into bilirubin in the liver. Bilirubin appears as dark green-brown globules, in either intracellular or extracellular sites. Bile pigment is easily identified when present in canaliculi, but in intracellular sites it must be distinguished from other brown pigments. Bilirubin is stained by periodic acid–Schiff stain (PAS) (diastase resistant), and is more definitively identified with the Gmelin reaction, which gives bilirubin a green color, or Hall's bile stain. Hematoidin is another bilirubin-related pigment present in areas of old hemorrhage, which appears as a bright yellow or orange pigment and is of variable composition.

Lipofuscins are lipochrome pigments that are typically found in older patients, atrophy, or chronic injury. They are a group of substances produced by the progressive oxidation of lipid precursors and are composed of lipid or phospholipid–protein complexes. The more common lipofuscins appear as fine yellow-brown granules with parenchymal cells or macrophages, particularly in the liver or heart. When there is heavy accumulation of lipofuscin, the granules appear coarser and resemble hemosiderin. **Ceroid** pigment is formed at an early stage of oxidation and large amounts may be deposited in the smooth muscle of bowel in the "brown bowel" syndrome. The deposition of ceroid is associated with decreased tocopherol (vitamin E) levels and may present clinically with mucoviscidosis, chronic peptic ulcers, chronic pancreatitis, or biliary atresia. Microscopically, the smooth muscle cells of the bowel contain gray to light brown granules. Fluorescence microscopy will bring out lipofuscin pigment. Special stains which demonstrate lipofuscin pigment include

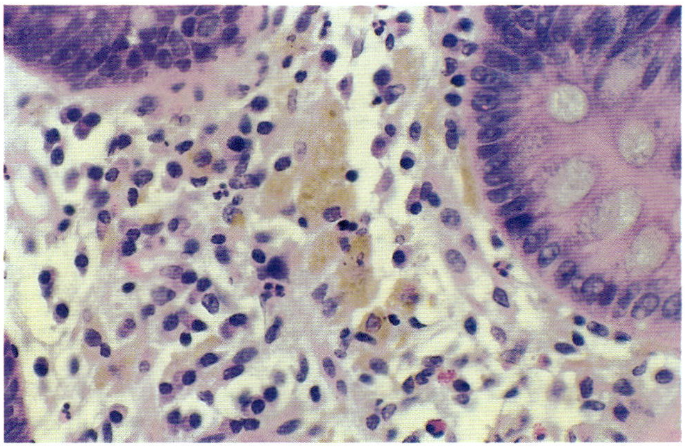

Fig. 6.5. Melanosis coli. Macrophages filled with fine particles in the lamina propria of the colon. The pigment is typically seen in patients ingesting excessive amount of laxatives containing anthrocenes.

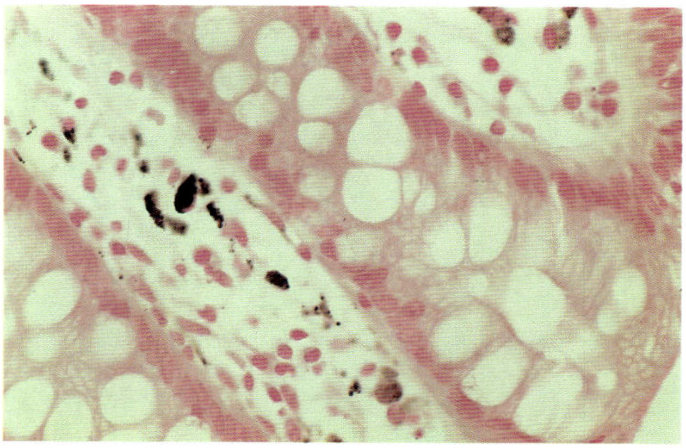

Fig. 6.6. Melanosis coli, silver stain. The pigment in melanosis coli shows positivity with silver stains, as well as PAS.

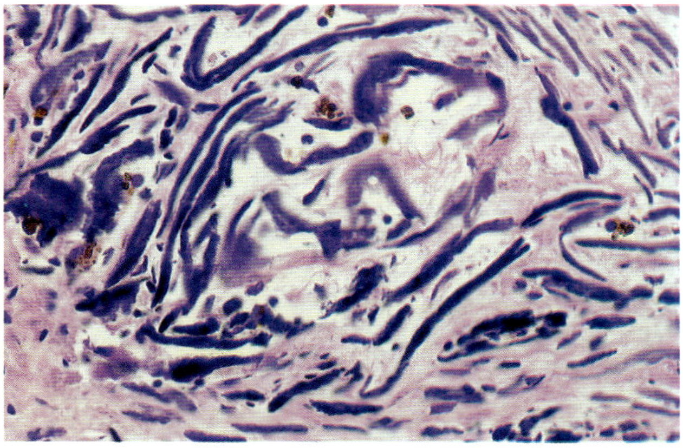

Fig. 6.7. Gamna-Gandy fibers, ovary. Gamna-Gandy fibers contain a mixture of iron and calcium and arise from the breakdown of hemosiderin.

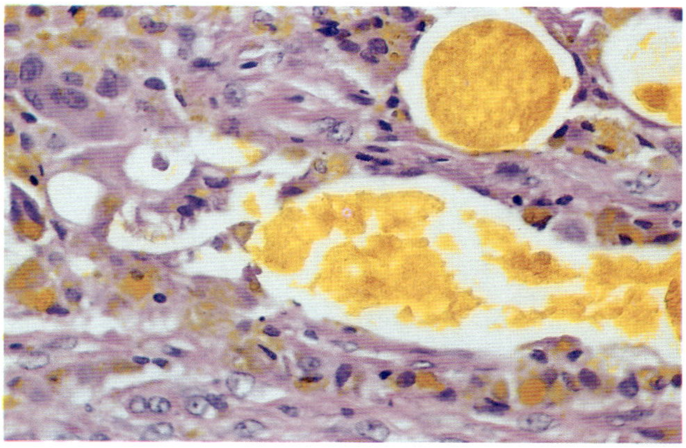

Fig. 6.8. Breast, biliverdin. The bright yellow pigment within macrophages and in the interstitium is a blood breakdown product. This patient had a prior excisional biopsy of a carcinoma which was reexcised because of positive margins.

Sudan black B, PAS (diastase resistant), Masson-Fontana, hexamine-silver slowly reduced, or modified acid fast (Fite) stains.

Prolonged administration of **minocycline,** an antibiotic related to tetracycline, may cause the thyroid to become grossly black (**black thyroid**). The same pigment has been described in the substantia nigra of the brain and in atheromatous plaques of patients on minocycline. The responsible pigment is most likely a mixture of neuromelanin and lipofuscin, since it stains positively with Fontana, is labile with bleach, iron negative, focally PAS-positive and acid fast stain–positive. On electron microscopic examination, the material appears to be contained in lysosomes.

Copper accumulation occurs in the liver with cirrhosis and is especially abundant in Wilson's disease (hepatolenticular degeneration). Copper is not easily visualized in routine hematoxylin–eosin (H&E) sections. Rhodanine and rubeanic acid stains are utilized to aid in the visualization. Coarse brown-red granules are demonstrated in hepatocytes with rhodanine stain. Protein is often associated with these granules and can be seen with orcein stain as purple granules in periportal and periseptal sites. Interestingly, copper in exposed sites may cause green color (oxidized state).

Homogentisic acid accumulation occurs in alkaptonuria (ochronosis). This metabolic disease involves the deficiency of the enzyme homogentisic acid oxidase. Homogentisic acid polymer appears as gray to black pigment, particularly found in skin, connective tissue, and cartilage. On H&E stain, the pigment appears as amorphous, smooth brown-black extracellular accumulations.

EXOGENOUS PIGMENTS

Carbon appears as a black particulate material, most often accumulating within lungs and its draining lymph nodes. Carbon is typically inhaled and is taken up by the macrophages of the lungs. From there, it can be transported through the lymphatic system, first accumulating within hilar lymph nodes (anthracosis). Microscopically, carbon is present in both intracellular and extracellular sites, as fine granules. Rarely, carbon appears in fibrous form in coal workers and patients exposed to wood stove dust.

During surgery, **India ink** may be injected into polypectomy sites in the colon, in order to aid the surgeon in the subsequent localization of a lesion. The ink is injected submucosally to form a bleb and subsequently may be seen from the serosal surface. Complications have included fat necrosis, inflammatory pseudotumor, abscess formation and peritonitis. Grossly, a blackened area is seen in the site of inking. Microscopically, the ink is usually diffusely present in the interstitium, and if it has been present for more than a few days, a chronic inflammatory response is seen. Desmoplasia may occur, with the formation of a fibrous nodule ("inflammatory pseudotumor"). The ink appears as minute black carbon particles, which coalesce to form aggregates within macrophages. Nuclei are obscured by the numerous granules of ink. Iatrogenic dyes have also been used to camouflage large hemangiomas, effective in deep lesions, but not so effective for superficial ones.

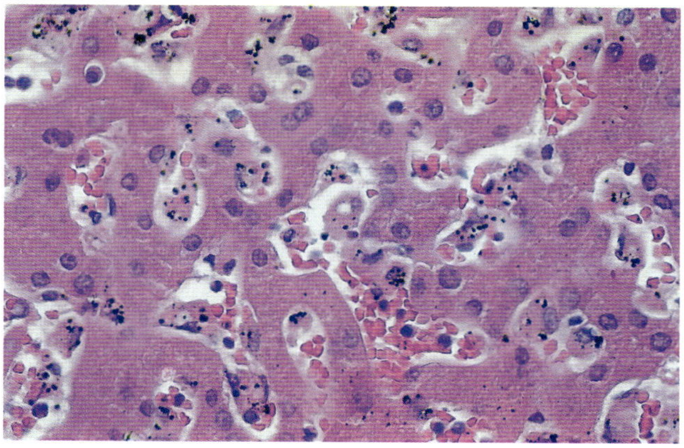

Fig. 6.9. Liver, malarial pigment. Coarse black granules are seen in the Kupffer cells lining the hepatic sinusoids from the breakdown of malarial trophozoites.

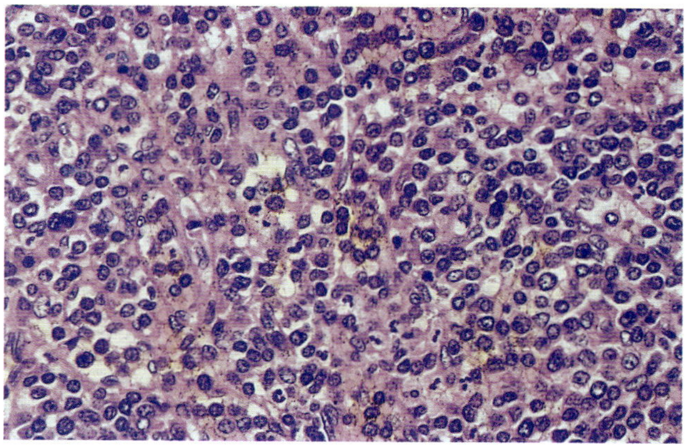

Fig. 6.10. Formalin pigment, spleen. Organs with large amounts of blood, such as the spleen, often show formalin pigment (acid hematin) after processing. It is similar to malarial pigment, but is extracellular and in a different plane of focus from the tissue.

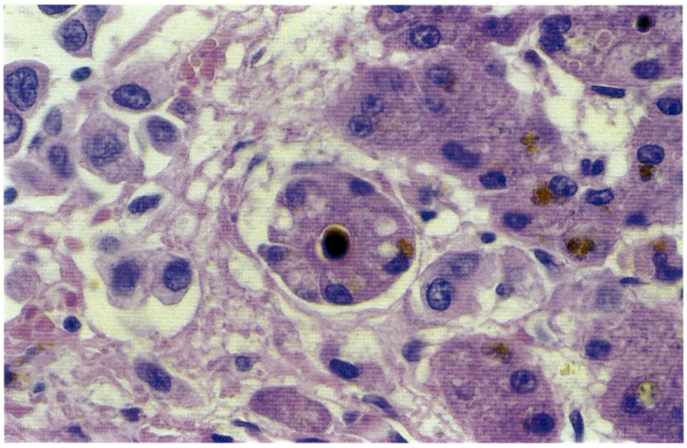

Fig. 6.11. Liver, bile. Bile pigment may be either intra- or extracellular, in parenchymal cells or in macrophages. It typically has a golden yellow to green homogenous appearance, without granularity.

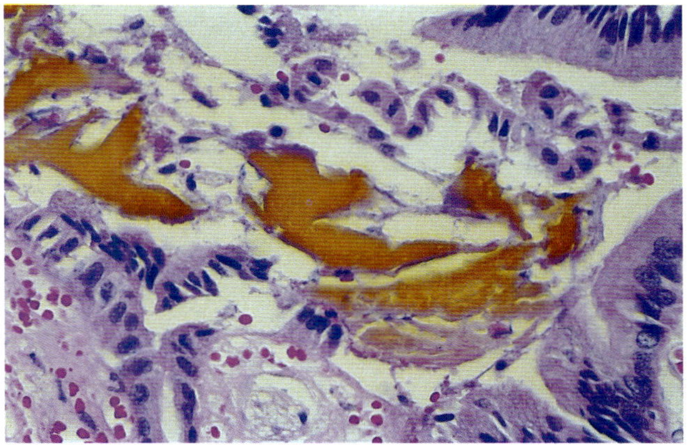

Fig. 6.12. Gallbladder, bile. This gallbladder retained the viscous bile fluid after processing. The bile is extracellular, present as large pools of yellow green material.

Inks are commonly used by the pathologist to mark surgical excision margins. The most common type is black India ink, but a variety of other permanent dyes may be used as well, including tattoo inks. Microscopically, the ink may be seen at the edge of sections, which is similar to the ink color seen grossly. If the ink is not quickly fixed, it may run into tissue crevices upon further sectioning. Dipping the specimen for a few seconds in Bouin's fixative or acetic acid will decrease the running of the ink.

Tattoos of the skin are composed of a variety of dyes, and include those derived from plants (indigo), insects (cochineal insects), metallic compounds (carbon—black/blue, cadmium selenide—cadmium red, ferric hydrate—sienna, mercuric sulfide—cinnabar, chromium oxide—green, cobalt—blue, titanium dioxide—white, ferric oxide—yellow, ocher, sienna—green). Gross examination of the skin shows pigmentation in a variety of colors and patterns. Intact tattoos are almost never excised, unless there is an associated lesion or unusual host response. Microscopically, tattoo ink is present in the dermis as intra- and extracellular granules, with minimal cellular reaction. However, allergic reactions have been described: a band-like lymphoid response similar to lichen planus or a more florid lymphoid response, called pseudolymphoma. Immunohistochemical analysis of the allergic lesions has shown the lymphocytes to be polyclonal.

Some tattoos are not deliberately placed. For example, metallic particles may be taken up by contact. Silver may be present in the dermis after wearing silver jewelry, amalgam in gums after dental procedures, gold and mercury in other sites. Argyrosis may occur as gray-blue to black pigmentation of skin after therapeutic administration of silver nitrate for gastric ulcers. Exposure to light reduces silver compounds to colored silver.

IDENTIFICATION OF UNKNOWN PIGMENT

Most commonly, an unknown pigment appears as brown granules and may represent formalin or malaria pigment, hemosiderin, or melanin (Table 6.1). Polarization microscopy will identify hematin, which may be intracellular and localized (malaria pigment) or extracellular and diffuse (formalin pigment). Other fixation artifacts such as mercury or chromate are also extracellular and diffuse; they can be removed by their different solubilities. Next, an iron stain should be performed to rule out hemosiderin. If the iron stain is negative, a melanin stain (Masson-Fontana, melanin bleach) should be performed. If the substance is not melanin, PAS will identify lipofuscin. Other pigments are rarer and special stains can be performed after further attempts to obtain appropriate history.

The differential diagnosis of microscopically visualized pigment based on color includes the following. **Black** may be due to metal (silver, carbon, gold, etc.), melanin, tattoo, India ink (inkoma), or minocycline (black thyroid). **Red** pigments include tattoo inks and red blood cell fragments. **Yellow** can be biliverdin or tattoos. **Green** is the color of copper and of tattoos.

Table 6.1. Identification of Brown Pigment

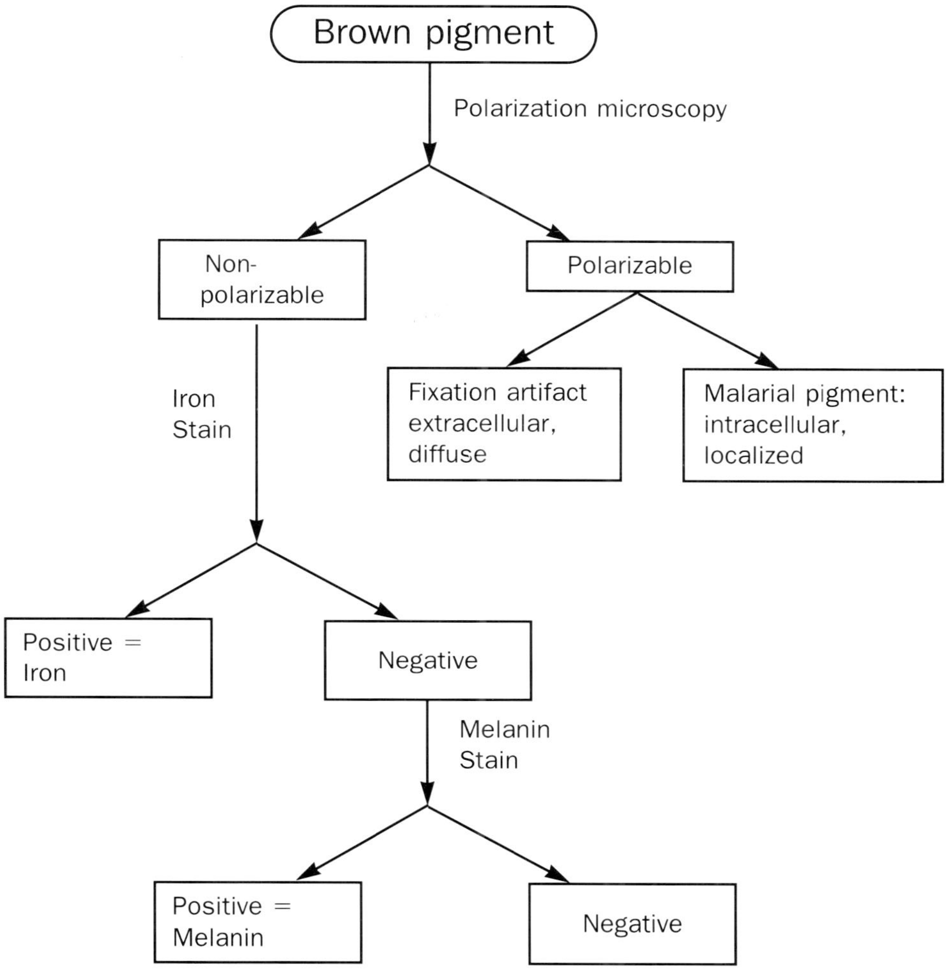

BIBLIOGRAPHY

Badiali D, Marcheggiano A, Pallone F, et al: Melanosis of the rectum in patients with chronic constipation. *Dis Col Rect* 28:241–245, 1985.

Blumental G, Okun MR, Ponitch JA: Pseudolymphomatous reaction to tattoos. *J Am Acad Dermatol* 6:485–488, 1982.

Coman E, Brandt LJ, Brenner S: Fat necrosis and inflammatory psuedotumor due to endoscopic tattooing of the colon with India ink. *Gastrointest Endosc* 37:65–68, 1991.

Fennerty MB, Sampliner RE, Hixson LJ, et al: Effectiveness of India ink as a long-term colonic mucosal marker. *Am J Gastroenterol* 87:79–81, 1992.

Food and Drug Administration: Tattoos. *FCA Med Bull* 24(1):8, 1994.

Fox B: Lipofuscinosis of the gastrointestinal tract in man. *J Clin Pathol* 20:806–813, 1967.

Goldstein AP: Histologic reactions in tattoos. *J Dermatol Surg Oncol* 5:896–900, 1979.

Hyman N, Wayne JD: Endoscopic four quadrant tattoo for the identification of colonic lesions at surgery. *Gastrointest Endosc* 37:56–58, 1991.

Hytiroglou P, Domingo J: Development of melanosis of uterine cervix after cryotherapy for epithelial dysplasia. *Am J Clin Pathol* 93:802–805, 1990.

Krishnamurthy S, Schuffler MD, Rohrmann CA, et al: Severe idiopathic constipation is associated with a distinctive abnormality of the colon myenteric plexus. *Gastroenterology* 88;26–34, 1985.

Krishnamurthy S, Schuffler MD: Pathology of neuromuscular disorders of the small intestine and colon. *Gastroenterology* 93:610–639, 1987.

Loewenthal LJA: Reactions in green tattoos. *Arch Dermatol* 82:237–243, 1960.

Park SI, Genta RS, Romeo DP, et al: Colonic abscess and focal peritonitis secondary to India ink tattooing of the colon. *Gastrointest Endosc* 37:68–71, 1991.

Rijlaarsdam JU, Bruynzeel DP, Vos W, et al: Immunohistochemical studies of lymphadenosis benigna cutis occurring in a tattoo. *Am J Dermatopathol* 10:518–523, 1988.

Shatz BA, Thavorides V: Colonic tattoo for follow-up of endoscopic sessile polypectomy. *Gastrointest Endosc* 37:59–60, 1991.

Schnitzer B, Loessel LS: Brown bowel. *Am J Clin Pathol* 50:433–439, 1968.

Smith B: Pathologic changes in the colon produced by anthraquinone purgatives. *Dis Col Rect* 16:455–458, 1973.

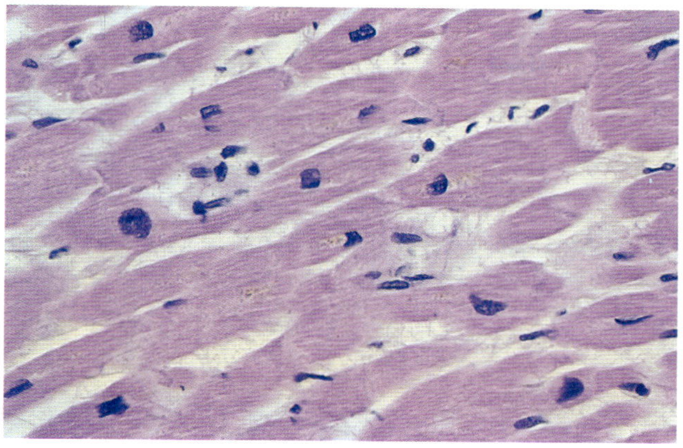

Fig. 6.13. Heart, lipofuscin. Lipofuscin, known as the aging pigment, is seen in a variety of organs with increasing age. It appears as intracellular yellow brown granules.

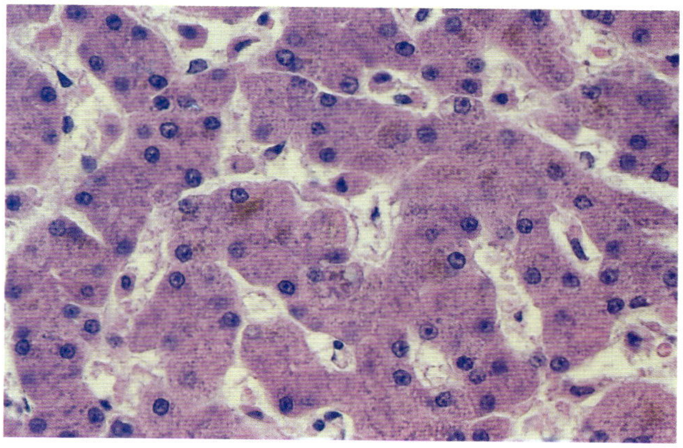

Fig. 6.14. Liver, lipofuscin. Compared with hemosiderin (Figure 6.3), the granules of lipofuscin are lighter yellow and finer.

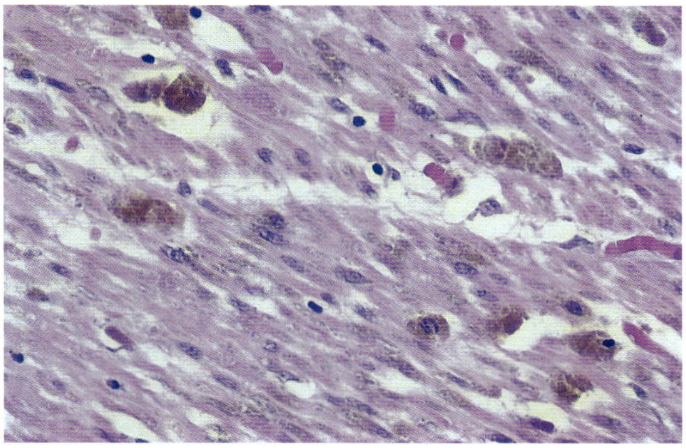

Fig. 6.15. Small bowel muscle, ceroid. This patient presented with the "brown bowel" syndrome and shows ceroid within the smooth muscle cells of the small bowel. Ceroid is basically the same as lipofuscin and shows similar staining characteristics.

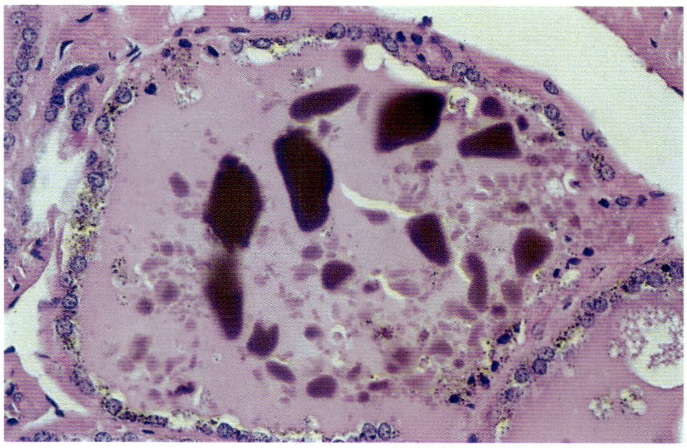

Fig. 6.16. Black thyroid. The patient was treated with long-term minocycline therapy. Numerous black granules within thyroid follicular cells, as well as gray-black pigmented areas of colloid are seen.

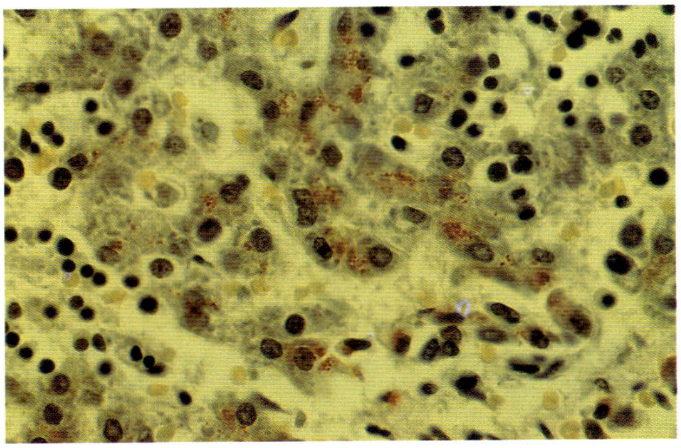

Fig. 6.17. Liver, copper, rhodanine stain. Excess copper accumulation was present within liver parenchymal cells in this patient with Wilson's disease. Copper granules were not easily visualized on the H&E stain, but are quite obvious on this rhodanine-stained section.

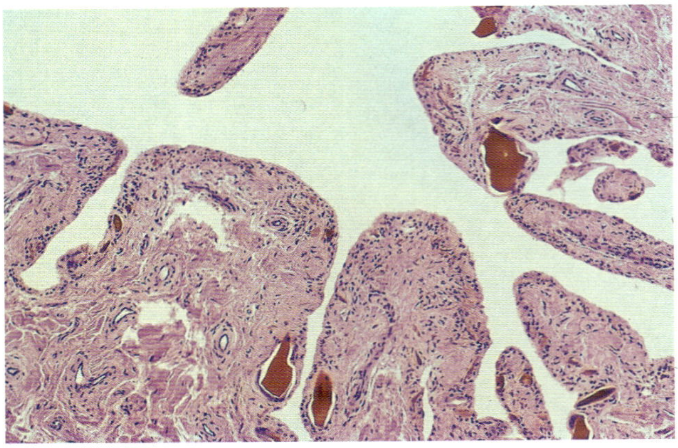

Fig. 6.18. Synovium, ochronosis. Low-power micrograph shows synovial proliferation in a papillary pattern, with gray-brown pigmented deposits of homogentisic acid.

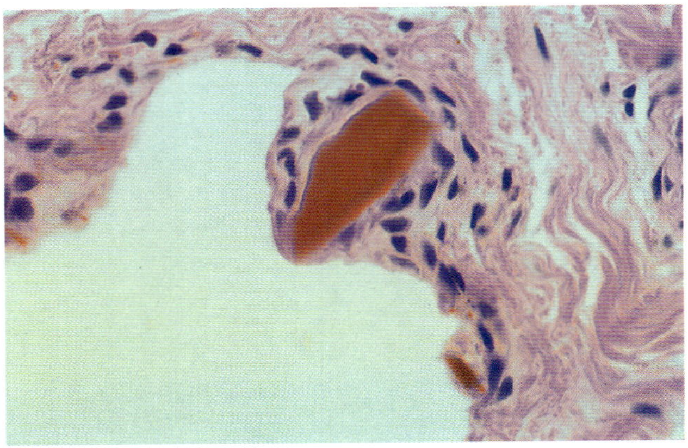

Fig. 6.19. Synovium, ochronosis. Higher power of the prior specimen reveals that homogentisic acid accumulates as amorphous extracellular deposits.

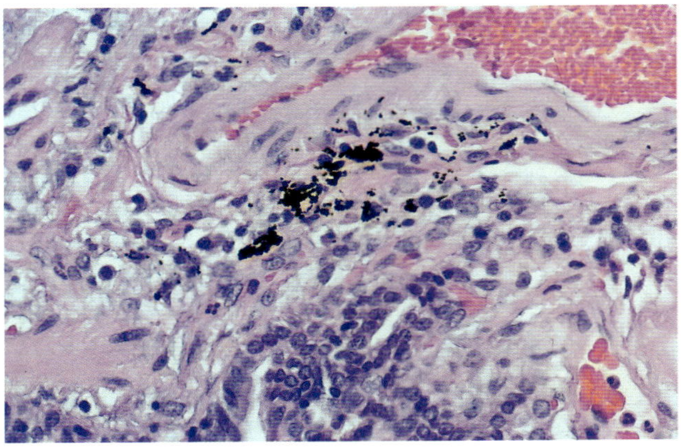

Fig. 6.20. Lung, carbon. This patient was an inhabitant of a city and inhaled carbon pigment. Carbon is present as both intra- and extracellular sites as fine black particles.

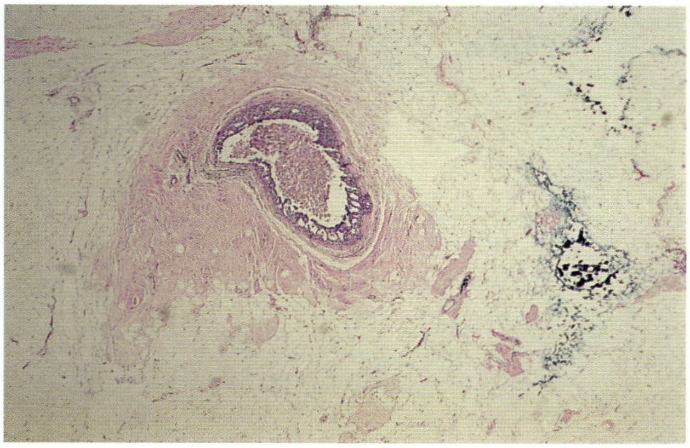

Fig. 6.21. Ink at surgical margin. This breast specimen contains an intraductal carcinoma that extends to the resection margin, which can be identified by the blue ink painted on the external surface of the specimen by the pathologist.

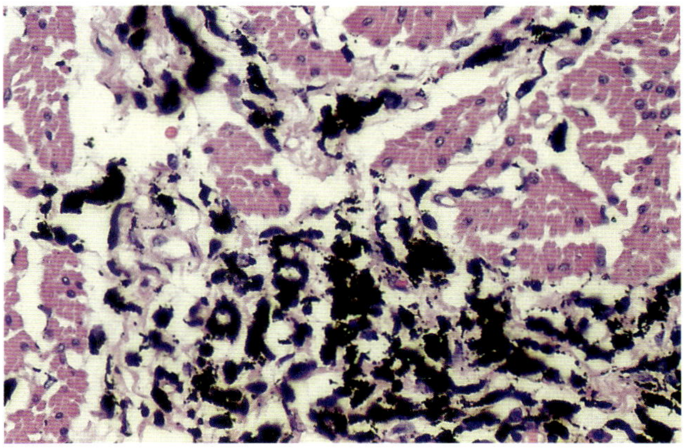

Fig. 6.22. India ink in esophagus, in site of adenocarcinoma. The tumor was a small superficial lesion which could not be easily palpated from the external surface. India ink was injected deep into the muscular layer to enable the surgeon to visualize the site for excision. Ink is seen separating muscle fibers.

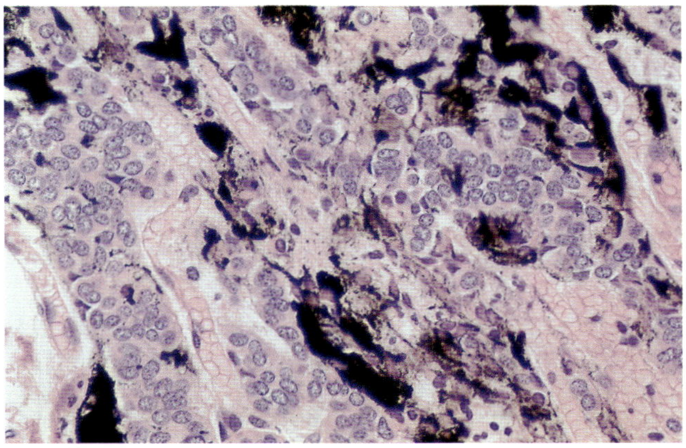

Fig. 6.23. India ink in carcinoid tumor. The ink was injected at the time of endoscopy, so that the tumor could be easily grossly visualized at surgery. The ink is in both intra- and extracellular locations and appears as minute black granules that may coalesce.

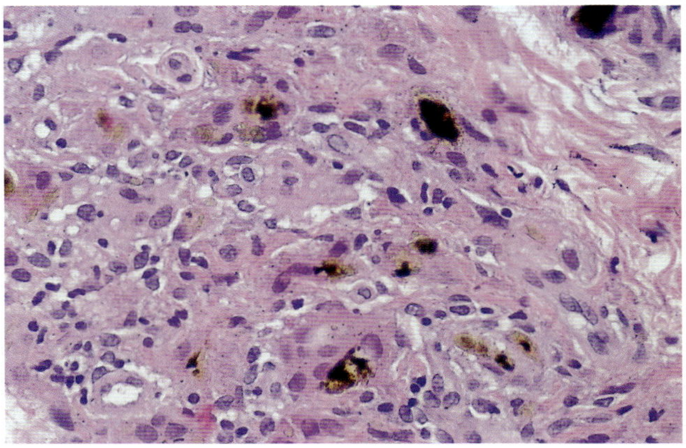

Fig. 6.24. Amalgam incorporated into gum tissue in a patient after a dental procedure. Irregular large black granules are present within histiocytes and giant cells as well as in extracellular locations. The granules vary in size from less than a micron to over 50 μm.

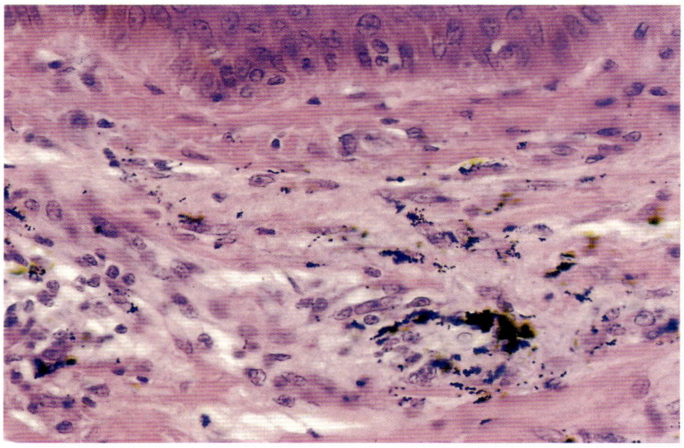

Fig. 6.25. Tattoo, skin. Dark coarse granules in histiocytes and in extracellular sites of the dermis are seen.

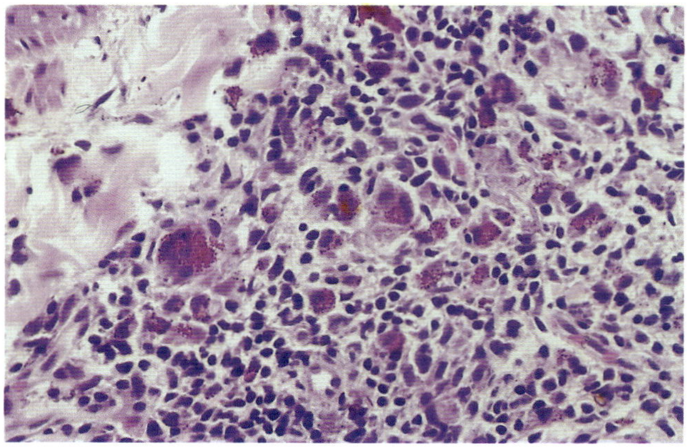

Fig. 6.26. Tattoo (red), skin. Coarse red granules are present within the dermis, located both in histiocytes and in extracellular locations. There is a florid chronic inflammatory response in this case.

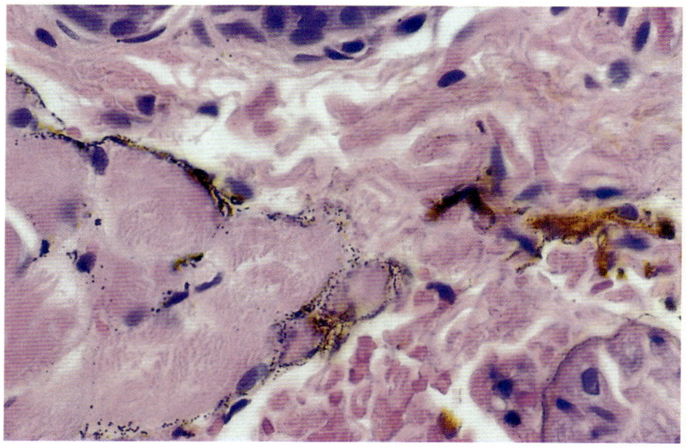

Fig. 6.27. Localized argyria, skin. Fine black granules can be seen either inside or outside cells within tissues exposed to silver, either from silver jewelry or iatrogenic applications.

7

Crystals, Crystalloids, and Radiologic Contrast Media

CRYSTALS AND CRYSTALLOIDS

Crystals are solid molecular structures in which the components are arranged in a periodically repeated pattern. The term crystalloid has been used to denote substances that have some characteristics of crystals. Many substances may crystallize, if ambient conditions permit the individual molecules to take up a regular arrangement. Formation of crystals occur when a crystalline compound becomes supersaturated, which may be due to increased solute concentration, pH or temperature changes. After supersaturation, a nidus needs to be present for nucleation of the crystal. Endogenous crystal formation involves exposures to surfaces, such as cell membrane fragments, collagen, or proteoglycan degradation products. Stasis bolsters crystal growth. If conditions are not ideal for crystal formation, the same substances may precipitate as amorphous accumulations. Unstable agglomerates may break and cause pathology; for example, calcium pyrophosphate shed from cartilage will cause synovitis; cholesterol emboli cause ischemia.

Some crystals are normal physiologic components of the human body, such as calcium apatite on collagen fibrils in bone. Other crystals are formed as a result of a pathologic condition: inborn errors of metabolism (cystine, leucine, oxalate), degeneration (calcium compounds), and atherosclerosis (cholesterol). Still other crystals may cause pathologic processes: lithiasis (obstruction), urate (inflammation), silica (fibrosis), and asbestos (neoplasia).

Identification of crystals may often be accomplished using only light microscopy, using knowledge of structure, color, and size. However, polarized light, special stains, scanning electron microscopy, x-ray diffraction, and other techniques may be necessary for definitive identification. Based on the organ site, a differential diagnosis of the likely types of crystals may be constructed (partially listed in Table 7.1)

Crystals may be proteins (amino acids), lipids, minerals, or combinations of compounds. Thus, many crystals are discussed in other chapters, particularly in the pigments, minerals and metals, and foreign materials chapter.

Protein and amino acid crystals include amyloid, whole immunoglobulin (Russell bodies), immunoglobulin light chains (Bence-Jones), cystine, tyrosine, and leucine, as well as proteins of mixed or unknown composition, such as prostatic crystalloids and crystals of Reinke.

Amyloid and immunoglobulin (including light chain) deposits are associated with multiple myeloma. Amyloid is not classically thought of as a crystal, but fits within the definition of crystal, since it is composed of regularly repeating units of either immunoglobulin light chain (AL) or nonimmunoglobulin protein (AA) in a β-pleated sheet. Deposits of amyloid are extracellular and appear as pale eosinophilic material around vessels or between cells. Light green birefringence is described when amyloid is stained with the Congo red technique. **Russell bodies** are round, blue to eosinophilic intracytoplasmic inclusions that may be seen in normal reactive plasma cells as well as neoplastic plasma cells. They vary in size, but may be quite large, up to several times the size of the usual plasma cell. When multiple Russell bodies are present in a cell, the cell can be called a Mott cell. In rare instances, the same immunoglobulins may crystallize into angulated eosinophilic inclusions.

Cystine crystals or calculi occur in patients with congenital cystinosis or cystinuria. In tissue sections, cystine crystals are small rod to rectangular yellow refractile crystals, located either in macrophages or in extracellular

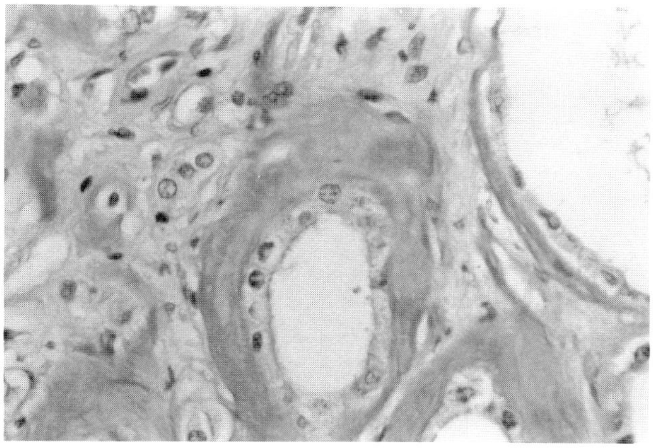

Fig. 7.1. Amyloid of kidney. Amyloid appears as a deposition of hyaline material around renal tubules.

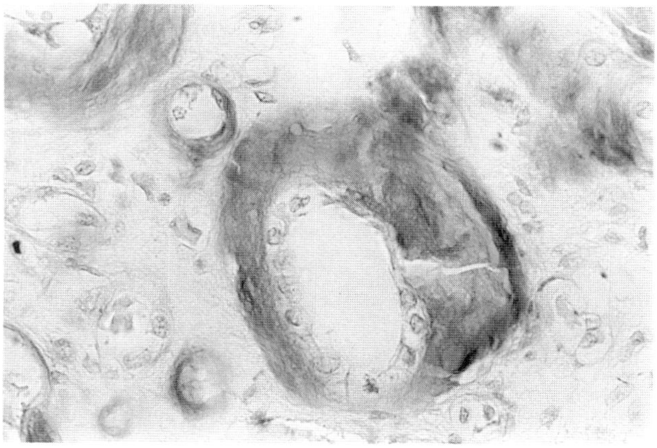

Fig. 7.2. Amyloid of kidney, Congo red stain. The condenser is turned down to emphasize the refractile nature of the amyloid. Marked positivity is seen as bright orange staining on routine light microscopy and "apple-green" on polarized light.

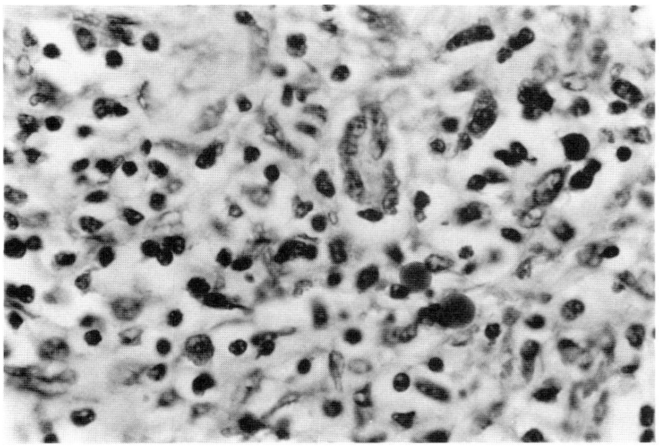

Fig. 7.3. Russell bodies. Spherical eosinophilic inclusions are present within the cytoplasm of plasma cells, which are infiltrating the interstitium of this renal tissue.

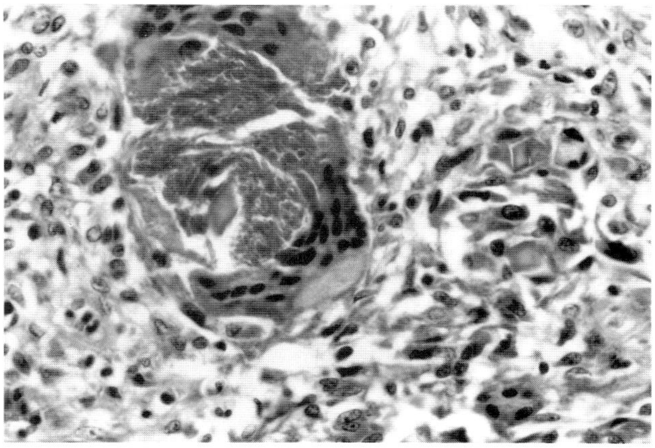

Fig. 7.4. Bence Jones crystals. Giant cells with rectangular, eosinophilic crystals are seen among more amorphous eosinophilic material.

Table 7.1. Crystals and Crystalloids by Organ Site

Bowel	Amyloid, antacids, barium sulfate, bentonite
Brain	Amyloid, calcium oxalate, corpora amylacea
Breast	Calcium oxalate, calcium phosphate
Eyes	Calcium oxalate
Genital tract	Calcium oxalate, calcium phosphate, crystals of Reinke, prostatic crystalloids, corpora amylacea
Heart and pericardium	Amyloid, talc
Hernia sac	Silica
Joints	Apatite, calcium pyrophosphate, urates
Liver and biliary tract	Bilirubin, calcium phosphate, cholesterol, silica, talc, thorotrast
Lymph nodes and spleen	Amyloid, calcium oxalate, cholesterol, cystine, immunoglobulins, silica, thorotrast, urate
Peritoneum	Apatite, antacids, barium
Respiratory tract	Asbestos, calcium oxalate, corpora amylacea, Charcot-Leyden crystals, graphite, radiologic contrast media, talc
Salivary glands	Calcium oxalate, tyrosine
Skin	Cadmium sulfide, chromic oxide, cinnabar, graphite, gypsum, iron, oxide, silica, talc, titanium dioxide
Thyroid	Apatite, calcium oxalate, calcium carbonate
Urinary tract	Apatite, calcium oxalate, calcium phosphate, cystine, leucine, radiologic dyes, tyrosine, urate

spaces. In urine, they appear microscopically as birefringent pale yellow hexagonal plates. Chemical identification is performed with the sodium cyanide–sodium nitroprusside test. **Tyrosine** crystals may be present in the urine of patients with liver disease, tyrosinosis, and Oasthouse urine disease. It is anisotropic and appears as haystack-like clusters of yellow-black needle-shaped crystals. **Tyrosine-rich** crystals occur as lightly basophilic aggregates in the myxomatous stroma of pleomorphic adenomas, a salivary gland tumor. They also contain tryptophan, arginine, and sulfhydryl groups. Like the urinary tyrosine crystals, a radial crystalline pattern is formed, but the periphery tends to have rounded, rather than sharp, edges. The Million reaction is positive. Crystalloids of the salivary glands may also be composed of amylase. **Leucine** crystals are found in patients with maple syrup urine disease, Oasthouse urine disease, or advanced liver disease. They may crystallize as plates, but are usually seen as yellow-brown globular crystals with striations.

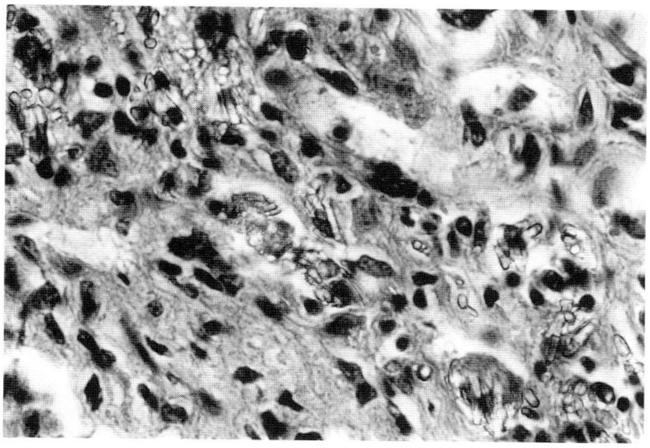

Fig. 7.5. Cystine crystals, kidney. This section of kidney is from a 2-year-old patient with congenital cystinosis. Numerous small rod-shaped yellow refractile crystals are present within histiocytes.

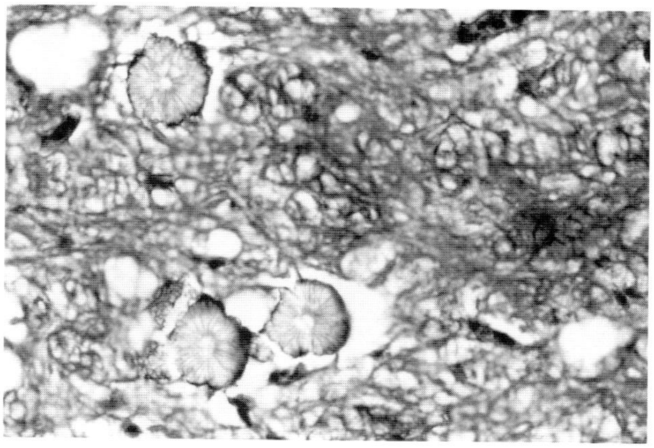

Fig. 7.6. Benign mixed tumor, parotid gland. Tyrosine-rich crystals are seen, characterized by clear, needle-shaped crystals radiating from a central point to form circular configurations within the myxoid matrix of the tumor.

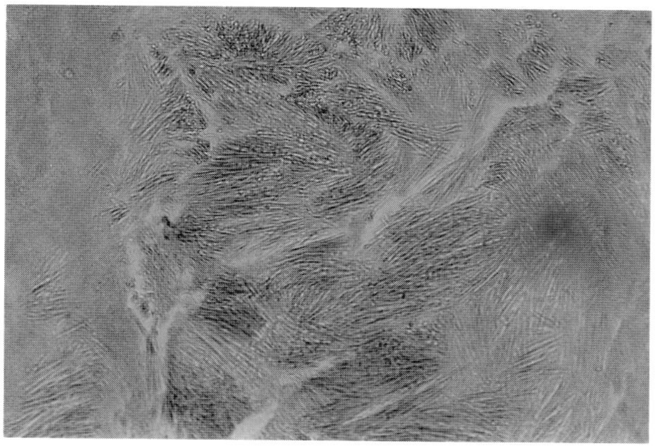

Fig. 7.7. Uric acid crystals, tophus. The crystals are seen in needle-like shapes, in clusters. Unstained sections or alcohol fixation will best demonstrate the crystals.

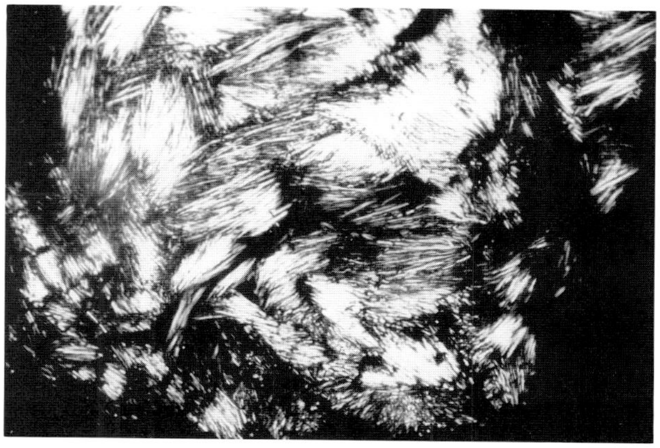

Fig. 7.8. Uric acid crystals, polarized light microscopy. Bright birefringence is seen.

Uric acid crystals are associated with gout, high purine intake, glycogen storage diseases, chronic nephritis, Lesch-Nyhan syndrome, as well as acute febrile conditions and tumor necrosis. In the examination of gouty deposits in tissues (tophi), urate appears grossly as chalky white soft material. Microscopically, uric acid collects in amorphous deposits, which are pale to light brown staining. Often there is a foreign body granulomatous response. With time, calcification occurs frequently. In the urine, uric acid crystals form in acidic conditions. Characteristically, uric acid crystals form diamond or rhombic prisms that may cluster together in rosette arrangements. Uric acid is markedly birefringent and may be seen in a variety of colors, partially depending upon the thickness and size of the crystal. These crystals usually dissolve on routine processing on tissue, but are preserved in alcohol.

Prostatic crystalloids are associated with prostatic adenocarcinoma but can occasionally be found in benign prostatic glands. These crystalloids are densely eosinophilic, extracellular (intraluminal) proteins, which vary in shape from rods to plates and even hexagons.

Corpora amylacea contain glycoproteins and may be found in the prostate and brain, as well as occasionally in the lung. They are typically extracellular, laminated, spherical structures.

Prostatic corpora amylacea are proteinaceous intraluminal deposits that stain a light eosinophilic shade and are usually seen in benign prostatic glands. The number of corpora amylacea increases with age, as does calcification of these structures. When large and calcified, they are essentially calculi, though prostatic calculi also originate from increased calcium and magnesium in secretions. Corpora amylacea are dichromatic with Congo red and metachromatic with crystal violet.

In the **lung, corpora amylacea** are found in intra-alveolar spaces, sometimes measuring up to 0.2 mm in size. They are also eosinophilic and laminated. Macrophages can be seen around the perimeter of corpora amylacea of the lung. Centrally, they can contain small black inclusions, which may be polarizable.

Corpora amylacea are present in benign **brain** as well. Although the designation is the same, they are distinct entities. The histologic appearance is similar to corpora amylacea of the prostate, but they are usually more basophilic. They tend to be located just under the pia or around vessels and increase in number with advanced age. Indications are that the composition of brain corpora amylacea is of glucose polymers, with only a minor protein component ($<5\%$). Thus, corpora amylacea of the brain stain with periodic acid–Schiff stain (PAS), iodine, and methyl violet.

Crystals of Reinke are found within the cytoplasm of normal Leydig cells of the testis, hilus cells of the ovary, but are more notable in tumors formed from these cells. Although these cells are known for their production of testosterone, a steroid, the crystals of Reinke are proteinaceous in composition. These crystals are rod-shaped, isotropic, and densely eosinophilic, ranging in size from 10 to 35 μm. They are usually single, but may accumulate in a parallel pattern. Masson's trichrome will stain Reinke crystals magenta, whereas iron hematoxylin will stain the crystals black.

Precipitated protein materials in more amorphous shapes include pulmonary alveolar proteinosis and colloidal micelles.

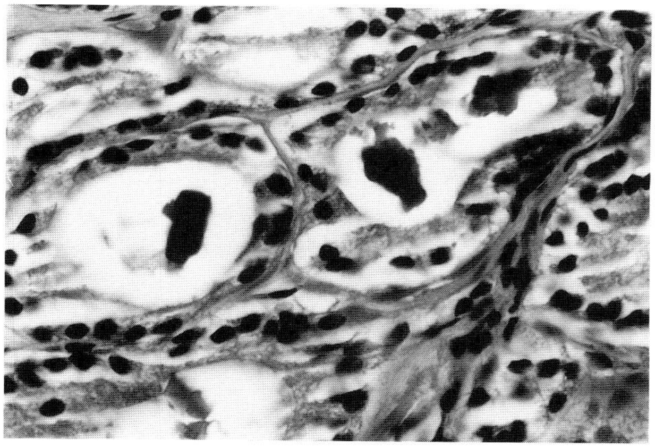

Fig. 7.9. Prostatic crystalloids, prostate. Angulated, intensely eosinophilic deposits are found within gland lumens in this well-differentiated prostatic adenocarcinoma.

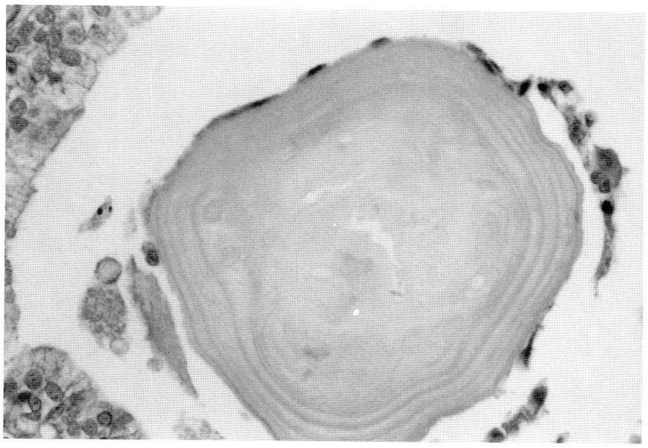

Fig. 7.10. Corpora amylacae of prostate. Concentric laminations of eosinophilic matrix are present in the intraluminal structure.

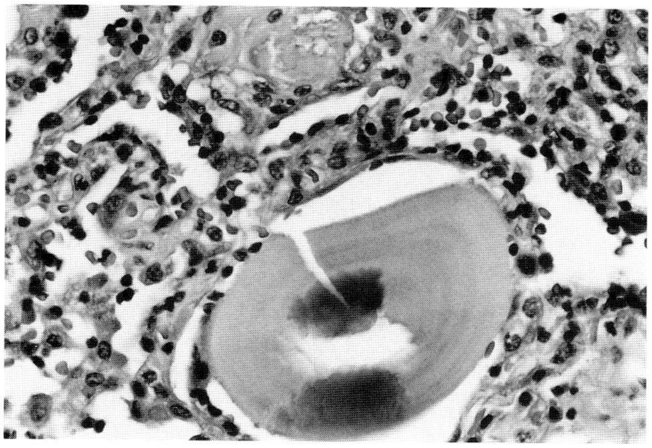

Fig. 7.11. Corpora amylacae, lung. These bodies are present within alveolar spaces, appearing as eosinophilic round to oval structures with concentric rings. In this case, there was some associated calcification that caused the section to be difficult to cut and a cracking artifact resulted.

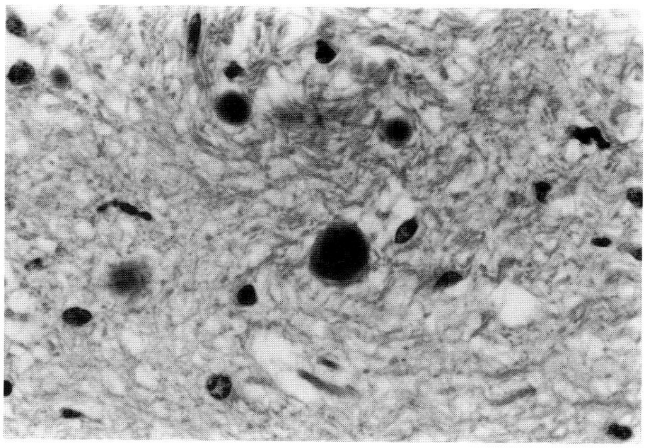

Fig. 7.12. Corpora amylacae, brain. In the brain, corpora amylacae are basophilic and appear in the interstitium as rounded concentrically laminated structures.

Charcot-Leyden crystals are bright red, needle-like structures with a widened center, formed of lysophospholipase, expressed by eosinophils and basophils. They are associated with asthma and other conditions causing eosinophilia, such as parasitic disease and neoplastic eosinophilic proliferations. Although typically extracellular when present in cytologic preparations, they may also be found within macrophages.

Crystals formed of **lipids** include **cholesterol,** as well as mixed lipids in **fat necrosis.** Common causes of fat necrosis include surgery, trauma, or pancreatitis. Routine processing dissolves lipids; therefore lipids are not easily identified with routine sections. However, the space that the lipid had occupied is preserved, and the presence of lipid can be inferred. For more definitive identification, the tissue must be processed without acetone, xylene, or chloroform. Oil-soluble dyes such as oil red O or Sudan black are useful. The most commonly observed lipid crystal is the cholesterol crystal, often formed from cell membranes in areas of cellular injury. In tissue, they are described as cleft-like spaces, either intracellular or extracellular, and vary greatly in size. In fluids such as bile or urine, cholesterol crystals are seen as colorless plate-like structures with notched corners. In its dissolved form, cholesterol is isotropic, but in its crystalline form, cholesterol becomes anisotropic.

Metabolic storage diseases with lipid accumulation include Wolman's (cholesterol ester storage disease), Gaucher's (glycosylceramide lipidosis), and Niemann-Pick's (sphingomyelin lipidosis), as well as many others. Histiocytes filled with the accumulated lipid are present in various tissues, particularly the bone marrow, spleen, and liver. While not always crystalline, these diagnoses should be considered in the differential of lipid accumulations.

RADIOLOGIC CONTRAST MEDIA

Prior to biopsy, a radiologic examination often is ordered; contrast media are frequently utilized to better visualize lesions. Those which are commonly encountered by pathologists include those media used in hollow organs, such as the gastrointestinal tract. Water-soluble contrast media are instilled into the bladder, uterus, as well as in the gastrointestinal tract.

Barium sulfate is routinely used as a contrast material in examination of the gastrointestinal tract. It may be found in the lumen, or if significant time has elapsed since the radiologic study, within macrophages of the lamina propria. In cases of ruptured viscus, barium may also be present within the peritoneal cavity, associated with a mononuclear or granulomatous reaction. Occasionally, barium is aspirated and found in the lungs. Grossly, barium appears as thick white material on the mucosal surface. Microscopically, barium appears as yellow-brown, strongly birefringent, coarse granules, either intracellularly within macrophages or extracellularly. X-ray diffraction studies on sediment after digestion of tissue in normal sodium hydroxide will provide definitive identification. A blue green flame will be seen if sediment burned on a platinum loop.

Of historical significance, **thorotrast** (ThO_2) is an α-emitter that was injected intravenously as for arteriography, particularly for the evaluation of hepatosplenomegaly. The half-life of thorotrast is 400 years, and deposits of this metal are accumulated in the spleen, liver, and bone, as well as other sites

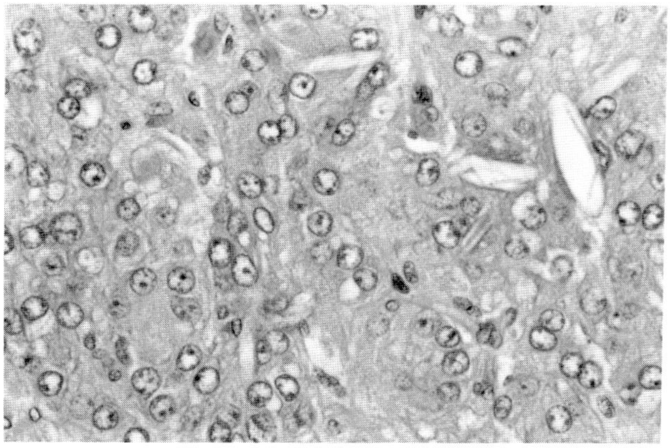

Fig. 7.13. Leydig cell tumor, testis. Crystals of Reinke are present within the cytoplasm of cells. They are eosinophilic and often appear in rod-like shapes within clefts.

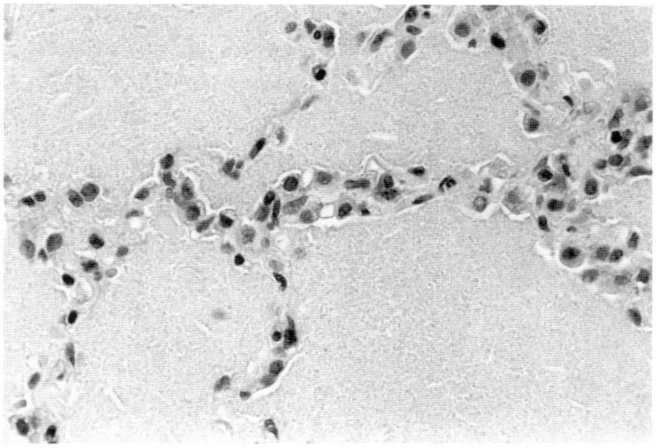

Fig. 7.14. Pulmonary alveolar proteinosis. Alveolar spaces filled with amorphous eosinophilic granular material. No distinct shapes are seen, as are typically seen with corpora amylacae.

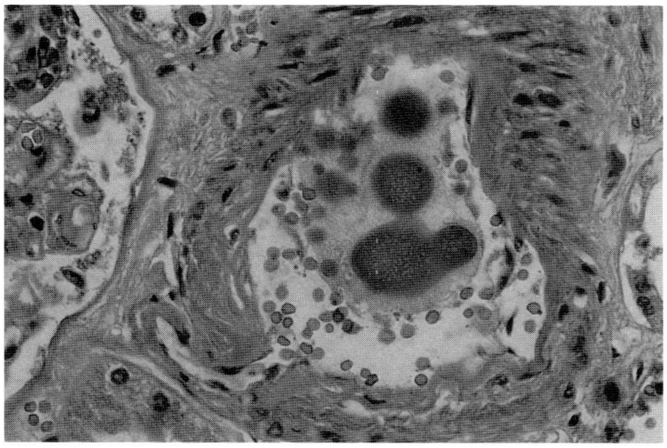

Fig. 7.15. Colloidal micelles. This patient died in shock, and at autopsy, colloidal micelles were noted with vessels.

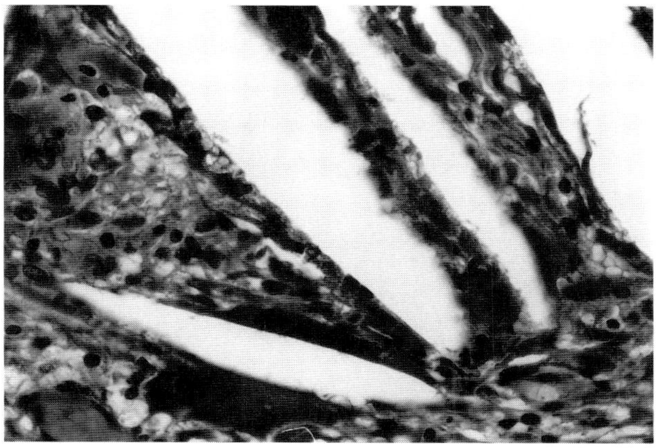

Fig. 7.16. Cholesterol clefts. This inflamed tissue shows large cholesterol clefts, surrounded by histiocytes and giant cells. The cholesterol has been dissolved by routine processing.

in the reticuloendothelial system. Thorotrast usage was associated with fibrosis, liver cirrhosis, hepatocellular carcinoma, and bile duct carcinoma. Since the 1960s, thorotrast has not been used due to these associations. No gross residual thorotrast is seen in contemporary specimens, but because of its long half-life, it is still seen in specimens from older patients. Microscopically, it appears as coarse light-brown to gray granules in reticuloendothelial cells or may be seen extracellularly in fibrous tissue. Thorium is isotropic. Quinalizarin stain will be positive for thorium; however it also stains beryllium, calcium, and magnesium.

The main substances to be differentiated from barium and thorium are hemosiderin and lipofuscin. Hemosiderin will be iron stain positive, whereas barium and thorotrast and are negative. Lipofuscin is PAS stain positive, and barium and thorotrast are negative. Definitive identification of thorotrast may be made by autoradiography or energy-dispersive x-ray spectroscopy (EDX). The characteristic birefringence of barium is not seen with either hemosiderin or lipofuscin.

Currently utilized contrast media include high-osmolality, **water-soluble, iodine-containing compounds**, such as diatrizoate meglumine and diatrizoate sodium (Hypaque, Gastrographin, and Renographin and iothalamate meglumine (Conray). Newer water-soluble contrast media may be of lower osmolality. Progressive dilution occurs as these substances move through the gastrointestinal tract. These substances are clear fluids, which may be dyed. Although soluble at body temperature, they will form white crystals upon cooling, and thus are typically crystalline in tissue specimens. These crystals may sometimes be visualized in urine after the patient had a radiologic exam with intravenous contrast. Formalin fixation and routine processing will wash out these crystals from tissue. The crystals are clear, relatively large, elongate rods, with blunt to pointed ends, appearing scattered or in irregular radial arrays, similar to a child's game of pick-up sticks. At times, more plate-like formations are evident. They are anisotropic on polarized light microscopy and are present in acid urine. The differential includes tyrosine, sulfonamide, calcium sulfate, and sodium urate. The crystals of radiologic dyes are usually larger and more distinct. A clue to the presence of radiologic dye is the high urinary specific gravity (due to the high osmolality of the contrast media). Low-osmolality, water-soluble contrast media do not precipitate as crystals under normal circumstances. Photographic development can be used to confirm that these crystals are radiologic contrast media.

BIBLIOGRAPHY

Agamanolis DP: The pathology of lysosomal storage diseases. *Path Annu* (pt1):247–285, 1995.

Bennett B, Gardner WA: Crystalloids in prostatic hyperplasia. *Prostate* 1:31–35, 1980.

Bowen JH, Woodward B, Mossler J, et al: Energy dispersive X-ray detection of thorium dioxide. *Arch Pathol Lab Med* 104:459–461, 1980.

El Okda M, Hyeh Y, Xie SS, et al: Russell bodies consist of heterogenous glycoproteins in B-cell lymphoma cells. *Am J Clin Pathol* 97:866–871, 1992.

Gomolin HI, Yamaguchi Y, Paulpillai AV, et al: Human eosinophil Charcot-Leyden crystal protein: cloning and characterization of a lysophospholipase gene promotor. *Blood* 82:1868–1874, 1993.

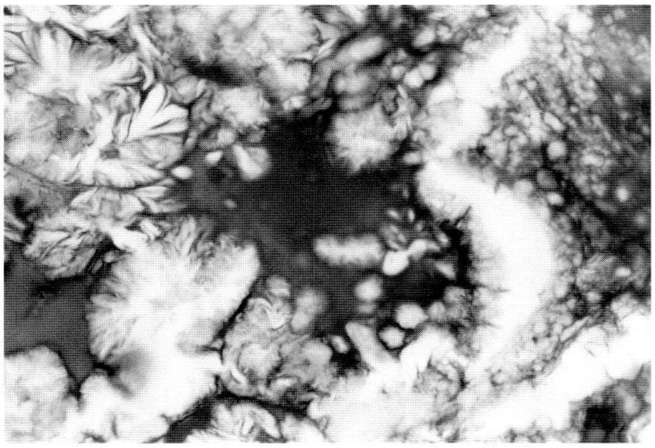

Fig. 7.17. Pancreas, fat necrosis. The necrotic fat contains needle-like crystals, which are composed of mixed lipids. These crystals aggregate in clusters, forming flower-like arrangements.

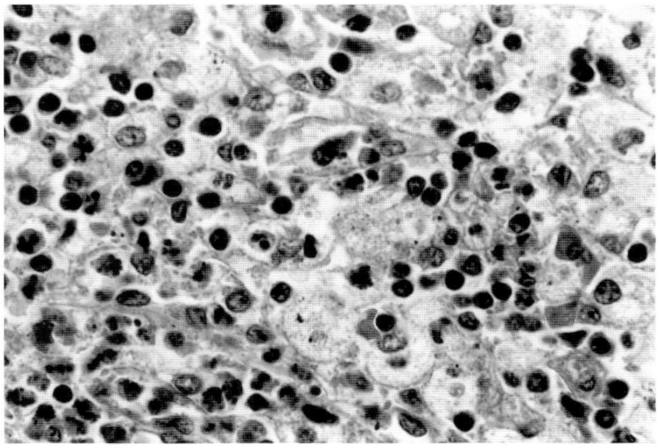

Fig. 7.18. Niemann-Pick's disease, spleen. Numerous histiocytes are present, containing sphingomyelin. The material appears foamy.

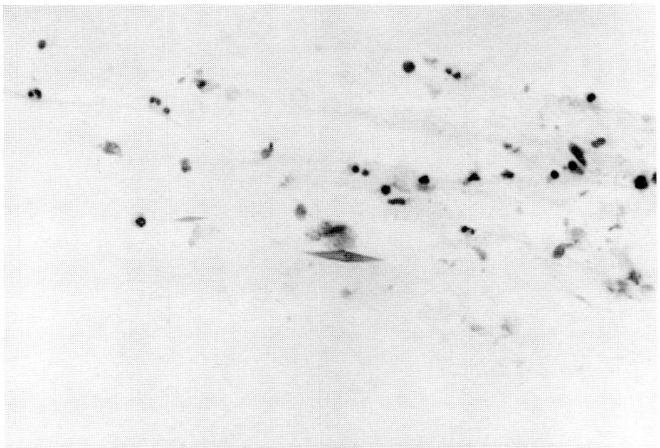

Fig. 7.19. Charcot-Leyden crystals, sputum specimen. A large angulated eosinophilic diamond-shaped crystal is seen among acute inflammatory cells, including numerous eosinophils (bilobed cells). (Photo provided by John SJ Brooks)

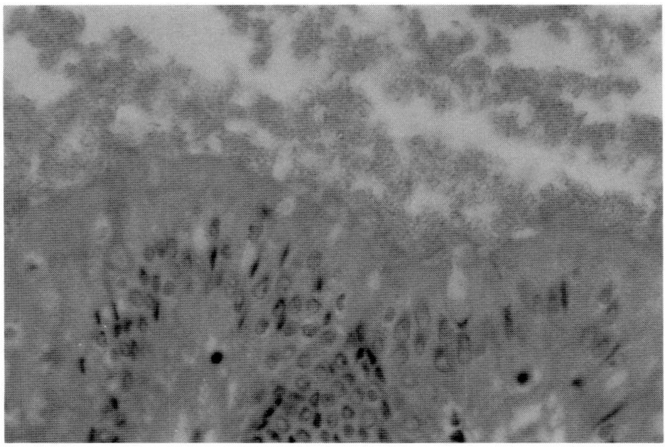

Fig. 7.20. Barium sulfate. Finely granular refractile barium is seen in the lumen of this bowel biopsy specimen (*top*).

Harris BR, Shipkey F: Tyrosine rich crystalloids in neoplasms and tissues of the head and neck. *Arch Pathol Lab Med* 110:709–712, 1986.

Holmes EJ: Crystalloids of prostatic carcinoma: relationship to Bence-Jones crystals. *Cancer* 39:2073–2080, 1977.

Humphrey PA, Ingram P, Tucker A, et al: Crystalloids in salivary gland in pleomorphic adenomas. *Arch Pathol Lab Med* 113:390–393, 1989.

Jenson PE, Gardner WA, Piserchia PV: Prostatic crystalloids: association with adenocarcinoma. *Prostate* 1:25–30, 1980.

Johnson FB: Crystals in pathologic specimens. *Pathol Annu* 7:321–344, 1972.

Johnson FB, Oertel YC, Ammann K: Sialadenitis with crystalloid formation: a report of six cases diagnosed by fine-needle aspiration. *Diag Cytopathol* 12:76–80, 1995.

Ro J, Ayala A, Ordonez N, et al: Intraluminal crystalloids in prostatic adenocarcinoma: immunohistochemical, electron microscopic and x-ray microanalytic studies. *Cancer* 57:2397–2407, 1986.

Rooney PJ: Hyperlipidemias, lipid storage disorders, metal storage disorders, and ochronosis. *Curr Opin Rheumatol* 3:166–171, 1991.

Saxe PA, Altman RD: Subcutaneous cholesterol crystals mimicking calcinosis cutis in systemic sclerosis. *J Rheumatol* 18:743–745, 1991.

Sugiyama H, Hainfellner JA, Lassmann H, et al: Uncommon types of polyglucosan bodies in the human brain: distribution and relation to disease. *Acta Neuropathol Berl* 86:484–490, 1993.

Wolf GL, Gazelle GS: Current status of radiographic contrast media. *Invest Radiol* 28(Suppl 4):S2–S4, 1993.

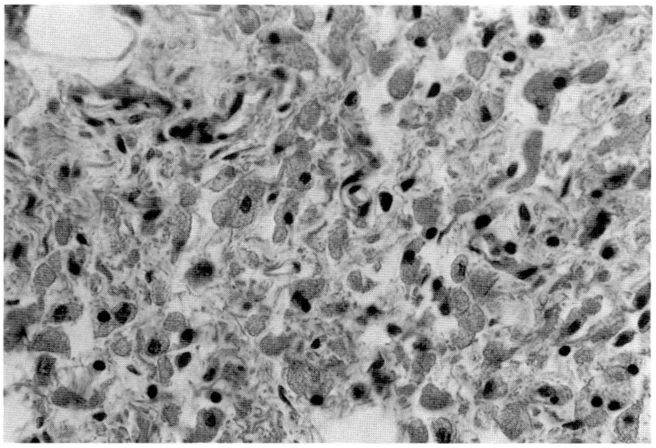

Fig. 7.21. Barium sulfate. Barium is present within histiocytes in the lamina propria of the colon after radiologic examination.

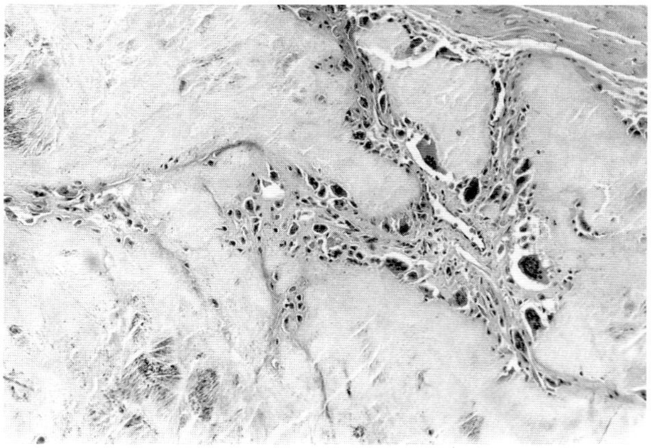

Fig. 7.22. Barium granuloma. Foreign body type giant cells surround the barium after extrusion of the barium from a viscus into adjacent soft tissues.

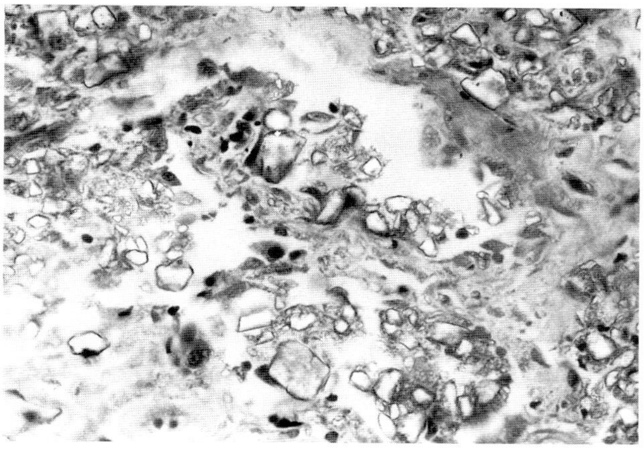

Fig. 7.23. Barium sulfate. Larger yellow-white angular crystals can sometimes be visualized. (Photo provided by Giuseppe G. Pietra)

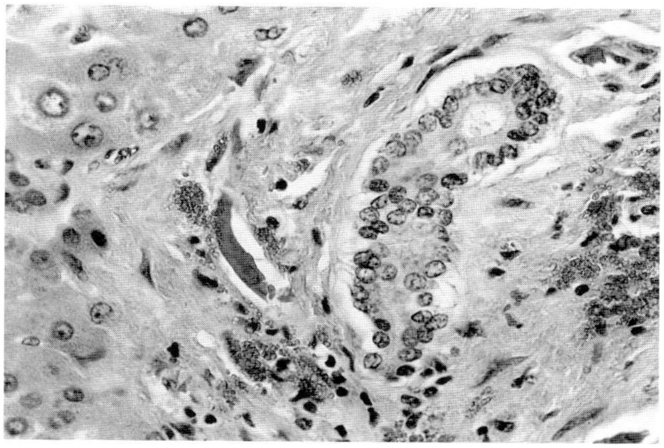

Fig. 7.24. Thorotrast, liver. The green-brown refractile granules in histiocytes around the portal area have irregular, slightly angular configurations. Many of the granules overlap and may obscure nuclei.

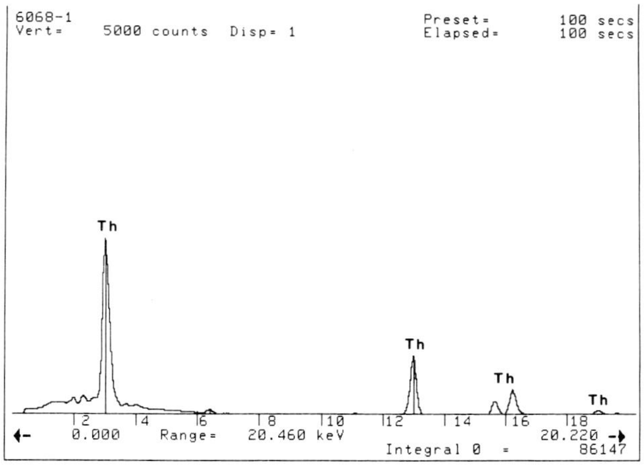

Fig. 7.25. Thorotrast, EDX. A prominent thorium peak is identified, confirming the presence of thorotrast. (Photo provided by Giuseppe G. Pietra).

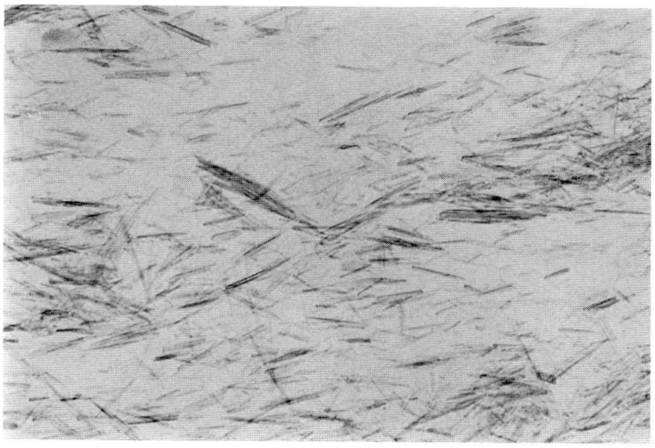

Fig. 7.26. Hypaque. Thin, rods, with pointed to blunt ends, mixed with amorphous material.

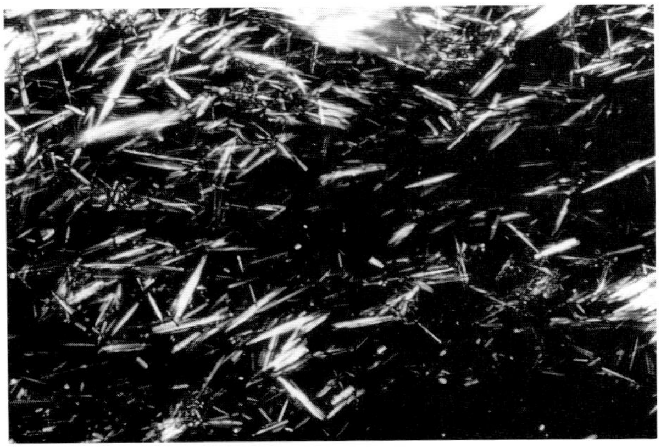

Fig. 7.27. Hypaque, polarized light microscopy. Bright birefringence is noted for the Hypaque crystals.

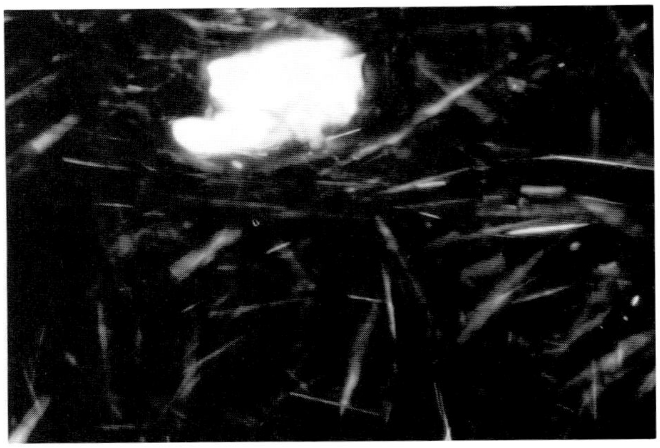

Fig. 7.28. Gastrographin, polarized light microscopy. Rod forms are mixed with more plate-like crystals.

8

Minerals and Metals

with Giuseppe G. Pietra, M.D.

In the complex industrial society in which we live, minerals and metals may find their way into human tissues by different routes, and the pathologist must decide whether these materials are "innocent bystanders" or have a role in causing pathologic changes. Few practicing pathologists have experience in material sciences and have access to specialized equipment to analyze minerals and other inorganic materials. Some clues to the identification of these materials in tissue sections can be obtained by histologic and histochemical stains or by examination with polarized light. However, precise classification is only possible by using microanalytical techniques such as energy dispersive x-ray spectroscopy. Energy-dispersive x-ray spectroscopy (EDX) requires an electron microscope equipped with an x-ray detector to capture the x-ray photons emitted by the atoms of a sample when it is hit by the high-energy electrons of the electron beam. The emitted x-ray photons are converted by the detector into electronic signals that are collected in a multichannel analyzer generating spectra that are unique for each element in the sample. EDX identifies only the individual elements present in a sample and it is not sufficient for the mineralogical classification of crystals. For this purpose, the identification of the crystalline structure must be made by selected area electron diffraction. The correct interpretation of diffraction patterns is not a trivial pursuit and requires considerable expertise.

Metals that are encountered in pathologic material include: titanium alloys, cobalt–chromium, stainless steel, lead, iron, barium, strontium, zinc, and aluminum. To identify the particular metal, the following methods may be used: histochemical reactions, microincineration, and electron x-ray probe. Histochemical staining methods are highly specific and sensitive. For iron, histochemical staining may detect as little as 0.01 μg; copper, 0.002 μg; barium 0.01 μg; and zinc 0.002 μg. Microincineration, used in conjunction with histochemistry, allows the localization and distribution of minerals. Analytical electron microscopy may be used to obtain quantitative information.

FIBROUS MINERALS

There is no scientific definition of fibrous materials. In general, a fiber is a single circular crystal or elongated polycrystalline aggregate having a circular cross section and a high length-to-diameter ratio. For regulatory purposes (OSHA), any object with a length-to-diameter ratio of at least 3:1 is defined as a fiber.

Asbestos is not a single mineral but a family of naturally occurring fibrous silicate minerals that share properties of great thermal and chemical resistance, flexibility, and high tensile strength. On the basis of physicochemical properties, asbestos minerals are classified as *serpentines* or *amphiboles.* Serpentines are composed of long wavy fibers, amphiboles of straight fibers of varying diameter. Chrysotile (white asbestos) is the best known serpentine and represents nearly 95% of the commercially used asbestos; crocodile (blue asbestos) and amosite (brown asbestos) are the only commercially important amphiboles. Other amphiboles, tremolite, anthophyllite, and actinolite, are widely distributed but of biologic importance only as contaminants. In histologic sections or filter preparations of digested lung tissue, asbestos fibers are optically clear, weakly birefringent, and may be straight or curved. Since most

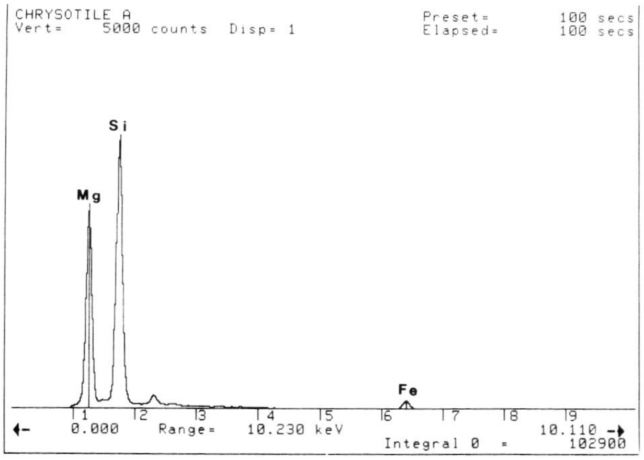

Fig. 8.1. Energy-dispersive x-ray spectrum of chrysotile asbestos. The photograph shows the typical x-ray spectrum of chrysotile that has the general chemical formula $(Mg)_6(OH)_8Si_4O_{10}(Fe+)$. The peaks in the x-ray spectrum indicate the relative proportion of the individual elements.

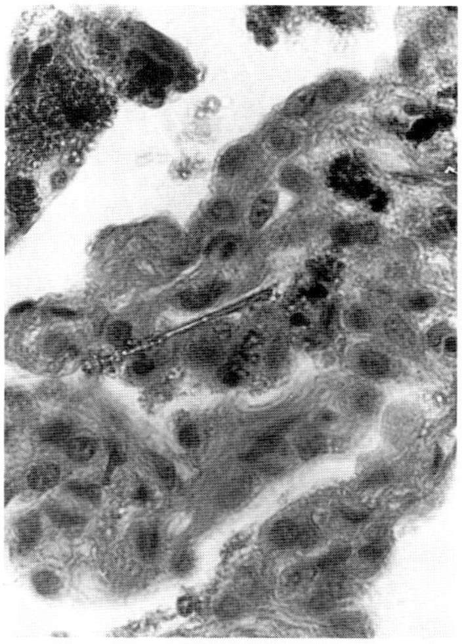

Figs. 8.2–8.5. Asbestos bodies. The appearance of asbestos bodies is heterogeneous. Asbestos bodies may have only a thin incomplete coat (Fig. 8.2);

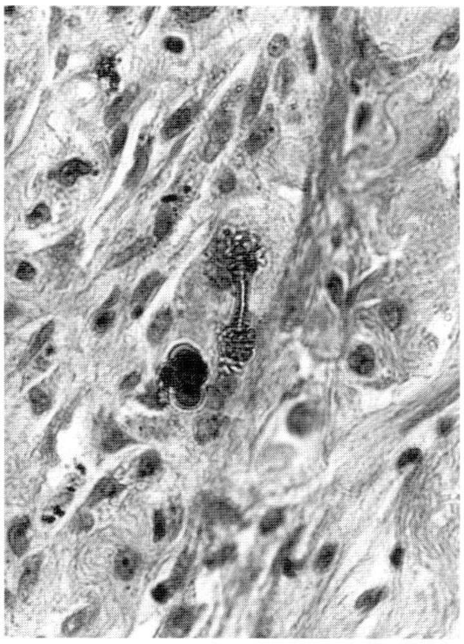

they can be straight with round ends (Fig. 8.3);

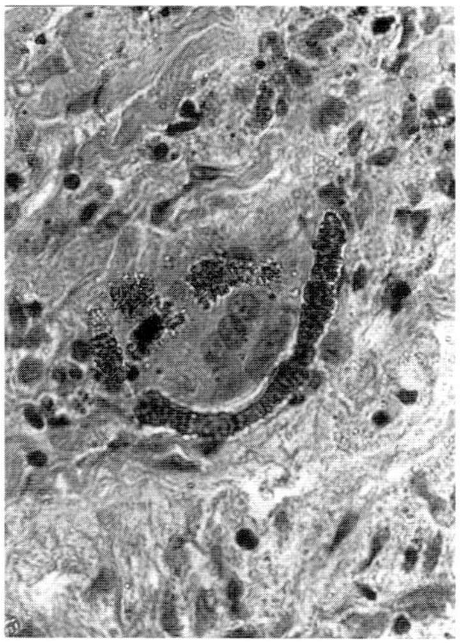

curved (Fig. 8.4);

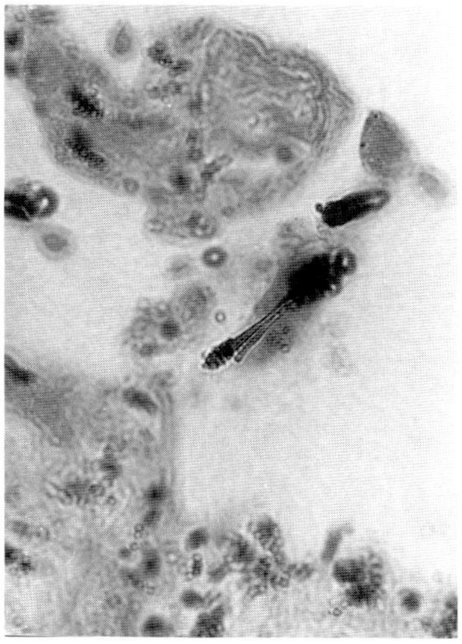

or split (Fig. 8.5).

asbestos fibers in tissue samples are below the resolution of the light microscope, they can only be detected by electron microscopy. However, only chrysotile can be identified as such by transmission electron microscopy because of its characteristic appearance of rolled up carpets when viewed in cross section. The precise identification of asbestos fibers in a sample requires EDX and selected area electron diffraction.

Asbestos bodies are long asbestos fibers, particularly amphiboles, that have become coated with a variable layer of protein and iron. Fibers coated with a variably segmented, golden brown ferroprotein layer are designated *ferruginous bodies.* Only those ferruginous bodies that have a thin, optically clear core have been shown to be asbestos bodies. Because of the iron content, an iron stain will usually be positive; however, occasionally the coating of the asbestos bodies may consist of calcium oxalate or calcium phosphate instead of iron–protein.

At the light microscopic level, the appearance of the core is helpful in distinguishing asbestos from nonasbestos ferruginous bodies formed on a variety of organic and inorganic dusts. However, when the core is masked by heavy ferroprotein coating, a precise identification is possible only by EDX. Ferruginous bodies formed on metal oxides (iron, titanium, aluminum, chromium) and carbon are characterized by thin, black cores. The core may be a hollow sphere (coal fly ash) or a solid and irregular particle (iron, carbon).

Silicates are common constituents of rocks, clays, and manmade fibers. Brightly birefringent fibers or needles are commonly found in the alveolar macrophages and among anthracotic pigment in adult lungs, particularly in cigarette smokers and urban dwellers. They are often confused with the needle-like crystals of silica which are only weakly birefringent and difficult to see in histologic sections. Silicates are often admixed with carbonaceous dusts' origination from burning coal in power-generating plants. The mineral inclusions in the coal fuse to form glassy aluminum silicate spheres (fly ash).

Talc is a hydrated magnesium silicate that occurs in sheet crystal easily cleaved into very thin plates. Commercial talc is rarely pure but is contaminated with asbestos, quartz, or carbonates. Talc used in cosmetic or pharmaceutical products is 90% pure and free of asbestos. Perivascular talc granulomas are now common findings in the lungs of intravenous drug abusers. Talc is used to create fibrous adhesions between the visceral and parietal pleura for the treatment of recurrent pneumothorax or pleural effusions.

CALCULI AND NONFIBROUS MINERALS

Calculi commonly form in salivary glands, the biliary tract, and the urinary tract. Calculi may be crystals or concretions, depending upon whether they are pure or mixed forms.

In **salivary glands**, calculi form in the milieu of an abundance of viscid mucus, alkaline pH, and stasis. The calculi have a layered appearance, due to alternating layers of organic substances (glycoproteins, lipids, mucopolysaccharides, cell debris) and inorganic minerals (calcium phosphate, calcium carbonate). They can be associated with infections, either as the cause or the result.

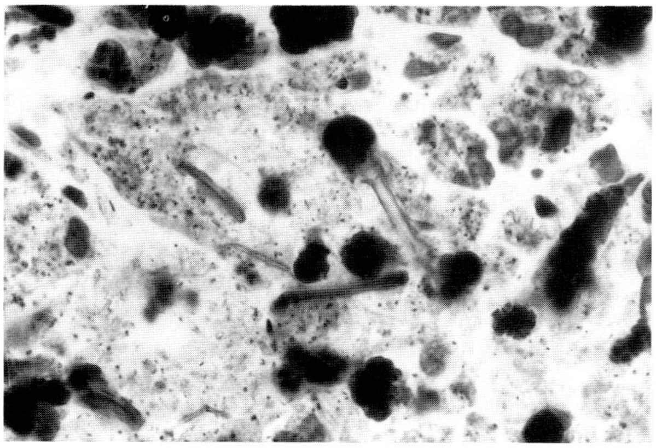

Fig. 8.6. Nonasbestos ferruginous bodies of the sheet silicate type. The microphotograph shows ferruginous bodies formed on talc (*arrowhead*). The cores of ferruginous bodies formed on sheet silicate (talc, mica) are broad, yellow, either fibrous or plate-like.

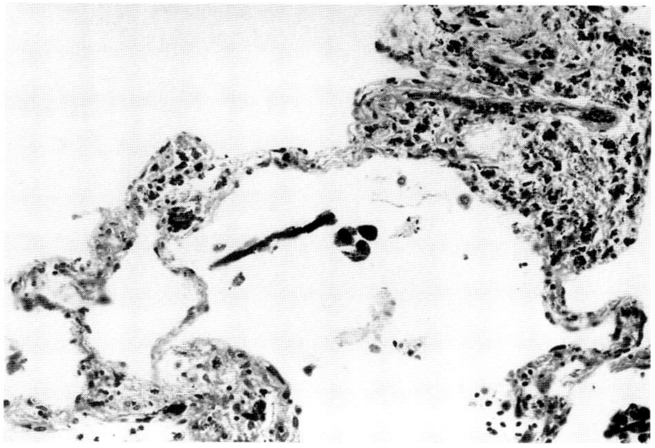

Fig. 8.7. Nonasbestos ferruginous bodies with dark core. Two ferruginous bodies with dark cores (*arrowhead*) formed on rutile (titanium oxide) in the lung of a metal worker.

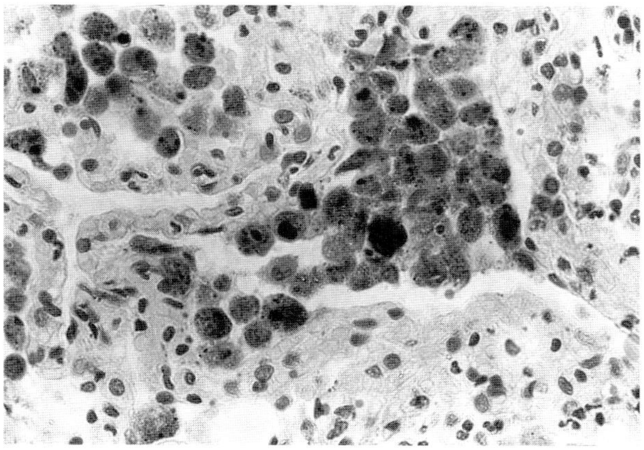

Fig. 8.8. Round ferruginous bodies. Nonasbestos ferruginous bodies may form on nonfibrous dusts and appear as round bodies with a black core (*arrowheads*).

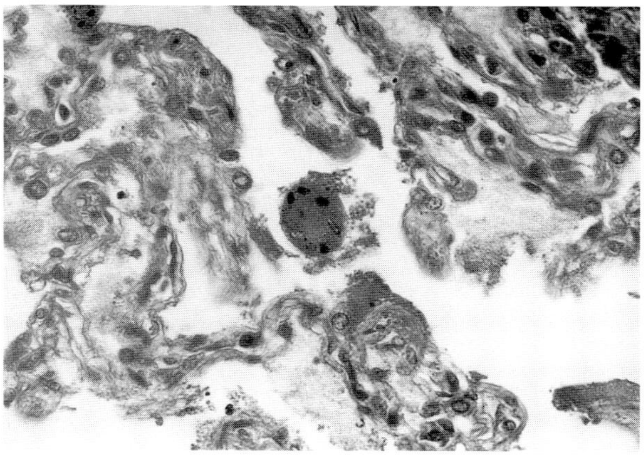

Fig. 8.9. Sheet silicates. Lung with intra-alveolar macrophage containing sheet silicate fibers (*arrowhead*).

In the **urinary tract**, calculi are often associated with *Proteus mirabilis* or *Ureaplasma urealyticum* infection, which both cause the urinary pH to increase, and thus magnesium and calcium salts to decrease in solubility. Abnormal crystals, including drug crystals, are typically found in acid urine. Other predisposing factors involve stasis, for example, due to obstructive prostatic hyperplasia, an indwelling catheter, or a spinal cord injury. Renal stones may be composed of a variety of elements and compounds, most frequently calcium oxalate, and many also contain phosphate and magnesium.

Within the **biliary tract**, a frequent cause of calculi formation is an increase in systemic solute concentration, such as hypercholesterolemia or hyperbilirubinemia. These conditions favor the formation of pure stones. Pure cholesterol stones are radiolucent, yellow-white, and round to oval in appearance. Cholesterolosis is often seen in the gallbladder mucosa in association with pure stones. More commonly, cholesterol is mixed with calcium and bilirubin. Mixed stones are faceted to round in shape, with variable coloration, depending upon the proportion of each component. Pigment (calcium bilirubinate) stones are less common and are associated with chronic hemolysis and cirrhosis. When pure, pigment stones are black, angulated and irregular in shape. They may be radiopaque (50%), are typically smaller than cholesterol stones ($<$5 mm compared with 20–40 mm in diameter), and form in sterile conditions, rather than associated with cholecystitis, as with cholesterol and mixed stones. If calcium bilirubinate is mixed with fatty acids, bile pigment calcium (brown) stones may result, which are brown in color, radiolucent, and have a softer, layered appearance. Infection of the biliary tract is invariably associated with brown stones.

Crystalline **calcifications** are typically composed of apatite, calcium oxalate, or calcium pyrophosphate. Apatite and calcium pyrophosphate are both compounds primarily composed of calcium and phosphate and are the common form of normal or dystrophic calcification. These compounds are sometimes found in virtually any tissue. Examples of these calcifications include granulomas, pulmonary blue bodies, tumors, sites of necrosis, as well as normal bone. Grossly, apatite appears white to brown, but may have different hues, depending upon the exact chemical composition, as apatite may contain other minerals such as fluoride or iron. As such, it sometimes stains positively for iron or carbonate. On hematoxylin–eosin (H&E) stain, calcium phosphate stains a deep blue. Apatite is isotropic. Although calcium pyrophosphate is similar in chemical composition, it is birefringent on polarized light microscopy. Alizarin red stains apatite but not calcium pyrophosphate.

Calcium phosphate (apatite) deposits in dead or degenerating tissues (dystrophic calcification) and in previously undamaged tissues (metastatic calcification) appear as concentric isotropic round masses that stain with varying intensity with hematoxylin and alizarin red. The deposits may also show an iron-positive rim and stain with PAS and Alcian blue indicating the presence of proteoglycan matrix. "Blue bodies" are dystrophic calcifications in the lung alveoli associated with a macrophage and multinucleated giant cell reaction. They appear as laminated oval blue concretions, which are variably sized, up to about 40 μm. Blue bodies will stain for calcium carbonate and calcium phosphate; thus both alizarin red S and von Kossa silver nitrate will be positive.

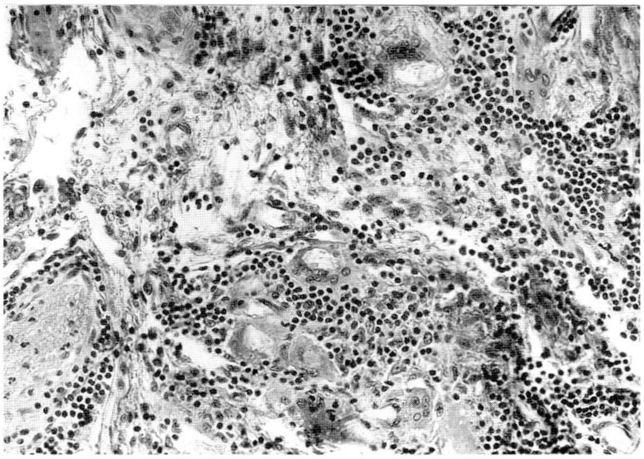

Fig. 8.10. Talc granuloma. The plate-like talc particles are strongly birefringent and readily identified within the cytoplasm of multinucleated giant cells.

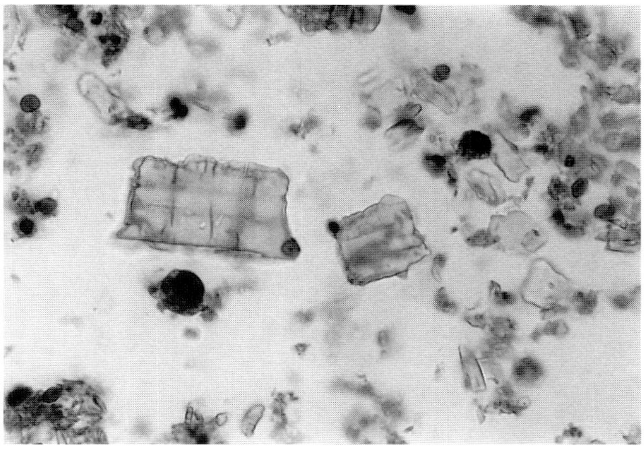

Fig. 8.11. Crystals, chronic sialoadenitis. Aspirated material contains numerous crystals which vary in shape and size from plate-like rectangles to almost round shapes. These crystals have a high concentration of amylase.

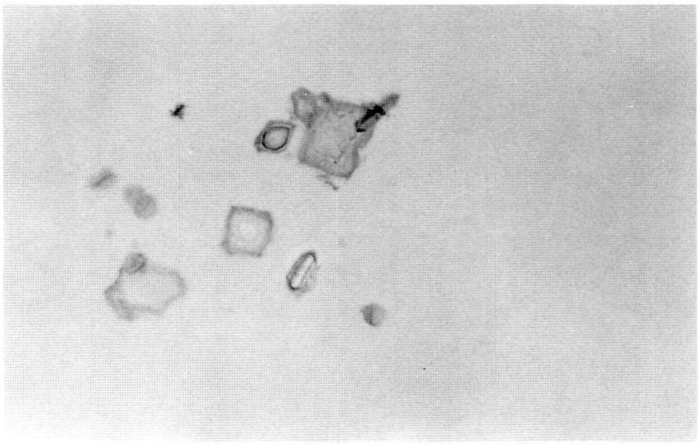

Fig. 8.12. Triple phosphate (ammonium magnesium phosphate) crystals, urine. Triple phosphate crystals are prism-shaped and clear, with 3–6 visible sides. They may be found in urinary calculi, chronic pyelitis, cystitis, and prostate hyperplasia.

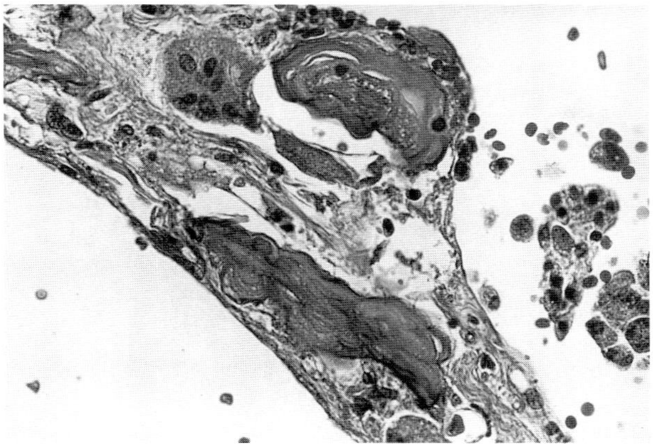

Fig. 8.13. Calcium phosphate (apatite). Dystrophic calcifications, in the form of intra-alveolar laminated concretions, are seen within alveolar spaces of the lung, known as "blue bodies." An associated giant cell and macrophage response is present. Although their etiology is uncertain, these blue bodies are typically associated with interstitial pneumonitis.

Calcium pyrophosphate deposits are found in synovial fluid, articular cartilage, periarticular soft tissues, and bone. The deposits appear in histologic sections as strongly hematoxylinophilic, alizarin red negative, layers of closely packed crystals without an inflammatory reaction. At low magnification, the deposits have a characteristic feathery or brush-like pattern, and the individual rhomboidal crystals can be recognized only at higher magnification. The birefringence of the calcium pyrophosphate crystals is much stronger in unstained sections than in stained sections. Definitive identification of calcium phosphate and calcium pyrophosphate deposits can be made by EDX. The x-ray spectra of calcium phosphate show a Ca peak greater than that of P, whereas the x-ray spectra of calcium pyrophosphate show equivalent P and Ca peaks.

Calcium oxalate deposits are found in patients with congenital hyperoxaluria or a variety of other disorders. Oxalate stones are at times associated with enteric hyperoxaluria due to fat malabsorption, such as jejunal ilial bypass for obesity, ilial resection, chronic pancreatic or biliary disease. A high oxalate diet can cause elevated urinary oxalate, since oxalate is a breakdown product of ascorbic acid, which can be found in such foods as asparagus, citrus fruits, garlic, rhubarb, spinach, and tomatoes. In breast tissue, calcium oxalate can produce mammographic calcifications that are associated with benign disease, which mimic the calcifications that are diagnostic of malignant disease. Grossly and microscopically, they are white or yellow and are irregularly birefringent. Calcium oxalate crystals are alizarin red negative in contrast to calcium carbonate crystals that are alizarin red positive. Calcium oxalate and calcium carbonate have the same x-ray emission spectrum; however, calcium carbonate crystals are dissolved by the Papanicolaou stain.

METALS

Beryllium is a highly reactive rare element extracted from beryl, a beryllium aluminum silicate. Beryllium oxide and several beryllium salts (fluoride, chloride, nitrate, and sulfate) are used industrially in the production of fatigue-resistant, lightweight alloys, heat-resistant ceramics, and "windows" for x-ray spectroscopes and x-ray tubes. Beryllium is highly toxic and may be absorbed in the lungs or the skin where it causes acute and chronic inflammatory reactions. From these sites, it is absorbed systemically and deposited in the liver, spleen, and bones where it may persist for a long time. Chronic berylliosis is characterized by the formation of non-necrotizing granulomas in the lungs, skin, lymph nodes, and other organs. Although the granulomas often show prominent Schaumann and asteroid bodies, they are usually indistinguishable from those seen in sarcoidosis. Detection of beryllium in tissue can be done in specialized laboratories using atomic absorption spectroscopy or electron energy-loss spectroscopy. Non-necrotizing granulomas resembling sarcoidosis can develop in individuals exposed to metal aluminum powder or to aluminum oxide. The epithelioid cells in the granulomas contain black round particles that by EDX consist mainly of metallic aluminum and aluminum oxide.

Systemically administered **gold** salts for treatment of rheumatoid arthritis may be deposited in various organs in the form of small, round nonbirefringent particles. The opaque gold particles are primarily intracellular, in the

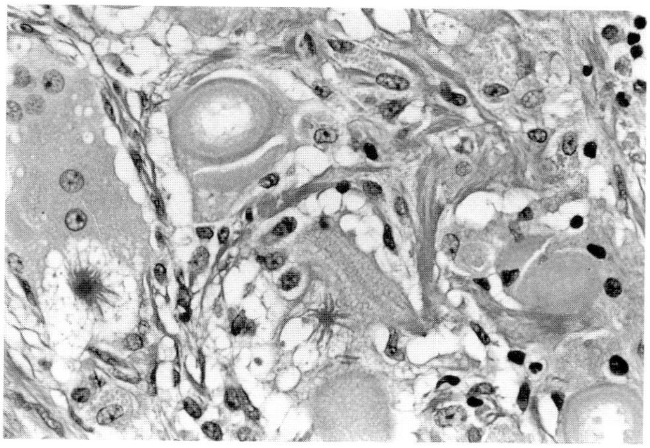

Fig. 8.14. Sarcoidosis, lymph node, calcium phosphate. These concretions may be up to 200 μm in size and are intracellular giant cell inclusions. Small calcium carbonate crystals may be seen centrally. At times the cells may rupture, and the conchoidal bodies may be present extracellularly.

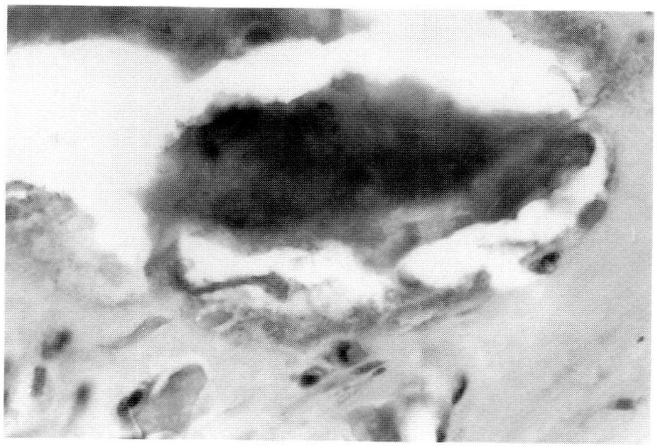

Fig. 8.15. Calcium phosphate, tumoral calcinosis, mass in trochanteric bursa. Grossly, the mass was gritty with creamy yellow areas. Microscopically, there are masses of amorphous purple acellular material, surrounded by fibrous tissue.

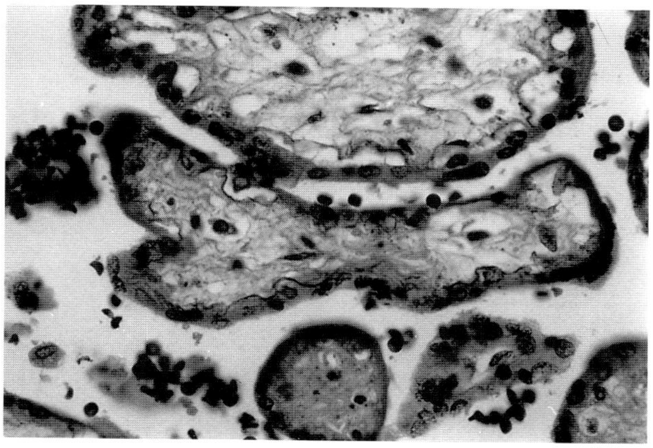

Fig. 8.16. Calcium phosphate, placenta. These placental villi contain linear deposits of basilar calcifications that are associated with senescence and/or fetal demise.

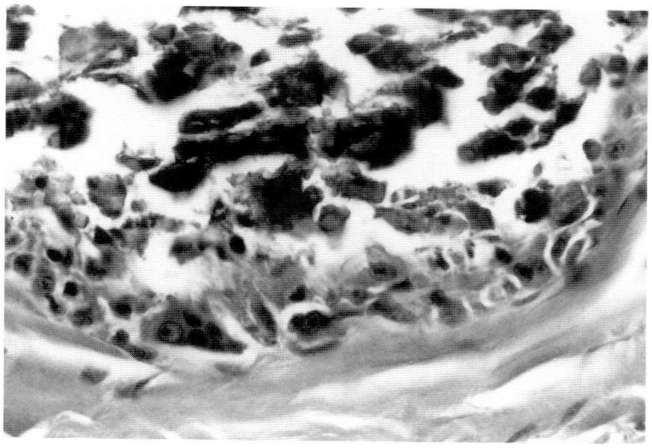

Fig. 8.17. Calcium phosphate, scrotal calcinosis. Irregular purple concretions, with giant cell response and peripheral fibrosis are present in this case.

cytoplasm of macrophages and in the periportal connective tissue, but they are not associated with a granulomatous reaction. EDX analysis will definitively identify the material as gold.

Black particles of **tungsten** (tungsten carbide cemented with cobalt) are found in the lungs of individuals exposed to hard metals, such as grinders, diamond polishers, and engravers. The resulting inflammatory reactions of giant cell interstitial pneumonitis (GIP) and desquamative interstitial pneumonia (DIP) are known as hard metal lung disease.

Iron-containing brown granules may represent hemosiderin or **magnetite**, a ferromagnetic mineral (Fe_3O_4). Oxogenous magnetite may accumulate in the lungs from inhalation of iron-containing ore (hematite, taconite), iron particles (grinders), or fumes (arc welders). In the lungs, exogenous iron deposits appear as heterogeneous coarse granules often with a central black core and admixed with silica. The alveolar macrophages of cigarette smokers also contain finely dispersed iron-positive cytoplasmic brown pigment, "smoker's pigment," that should not be confused with hemosiderin. Endogenous magnetite (biological magnetite) is found in many species ranging from bacterial to dolphins and humans. An ingenious, but destructive, method to distinguish between magnetite and hemosiderin is to place a suspension of chemically digested tissue on a glass slide located between the poles of a magnet before staining with Prussian blue. Magnetite particles align in parallel lines along the north-south poles of the magnet whereas hemosiderin particles are randomly distributed.

Mercury deposits are largely of historical interest, but may still be present in older individuals. Mercury was once the primary compound in glass fever thermometers, which were easily broken. Traumatic injury from the glass was not uncommon, with accompanying injection of mercury into tissues. In addition, mercury was a component of cosmetic creams, used to bleach skin. Chronic application sometimes produces brown-gray to slate-colored skin. Microscopic examination shows either a granulomatous response, in the case of traumatic injection, or fine irregular brown-black granules in the epidermis and superficial dermis, in the case of topical application. Mercuric granules are refractile on darkfield examination and definitive identification can be made by EDX analysis.

BIBLIOGRAPHY

Anttila S, Sutinen S, Paananen M, et al: Hard metal lung disease: a clinical, histological, ultrastructural and X-ray microanalytical study. *Eur J Respir Dis* 69:83–94, 1986.

Burge KM, Winkelmann RK: Mercury pigmentation. *Arch Derm* 102:51–61, 1970.

Crouch E, Churg A: Ferruginous bodies and the histologic evaluation of dust exposure. *Am J Surg Pathol* 8:109–116, 1984.

De Vuyst P, Dumortier P, Schandene L, et al: Sarcoidlike lung granulomatosis induced by aluminum dusts. *Am Rev Respir Dis* 135:493–497, 1987.

Dinsdale D, Bourdillon AJ: The ultrastructural localization of beryllium in biological samples by electron energy-loss spectrometry. *Exp Mol Pathol* 36:396–402, 1982.

Hall TA, Gupta BL: The application of EDXS to the biological sciences. *J Microsc* 136(pt2):193–208, 1984.

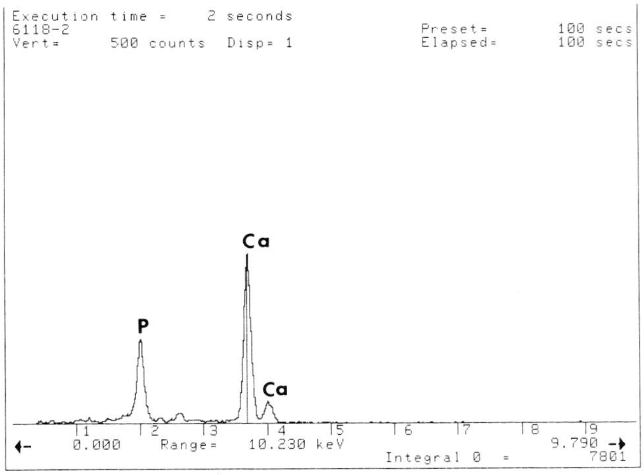

Fig. 8.18. Calcium phosphate, EDX. The x-ray spectra of calcium phosphate show a Ca peak greater than that of P.

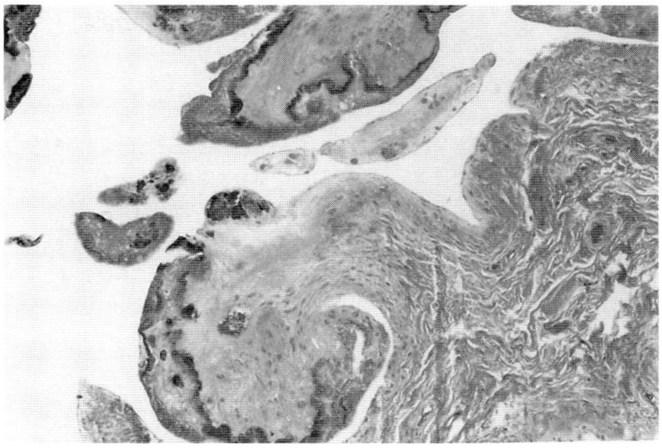

Fig. 8.19. Calcium pyrophosphate, pseudogout. This synovial tissue shows a calcified surface in a patient who had been treated with steroid injections.

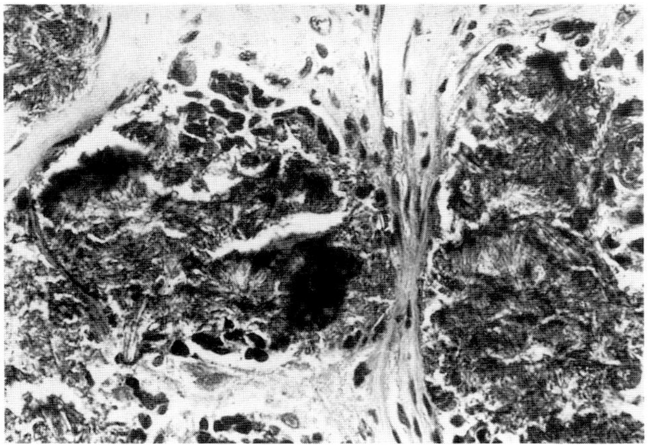

Fig. 8.20. Calcium pyrophosphate, synovial fluid. At low magnification, the deposits have a characteristic feathery or brush-like pattern.

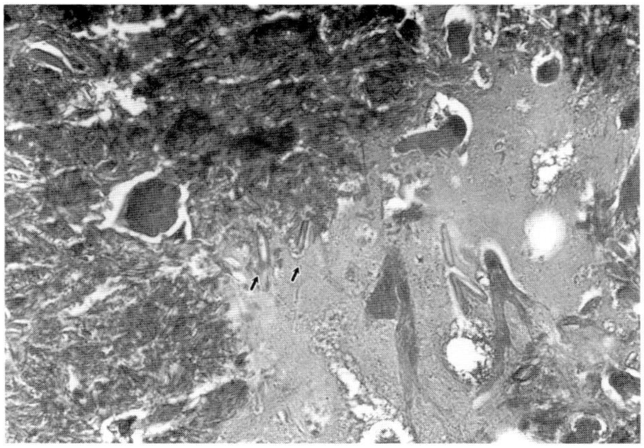

Fig. 8.21. Calcium pyrophosphate, synovial fluid. Individual rhomboidal crystals (*arrows*) can be recognized only at higher magnification.

Keen GE, Croker PR, Brady K, et al: Calcium pyrophosphate dihydrate deposition disease: morphological and microanalytical features. *Histopathology* 19:529–536, 1991.

Khan SR: Pathogenesis of oxalate urolithiasis: lessons from experimental studies with rats. *Am J Kidney Dis* 17:398–401, 1991.

Lamar LM, Bliss BO: Localized pigmentation of the skin due to topical mercury. *Arch Derm* 93:450–453, 1966.

Moatamed F, Johnson FB: Identification and significance of magnetite in human tissues. *Arch Pathol Lab Med* 110:618–621, 1986.

Ranki A, Nieme KM, Kanerva L: Clinical, immunohistochemical and electron-microscopic findings in gold dermatitis. *Am J Dermatopathol* 11:22–28, 1989.

Rollins SD, Craig JP: Gold-associated lymphadenopathy in a patient with rheumatoid arthritis: Histologic and scanning electron microscopic features. *Arch Pathol Lab Med* 115:175–177, 1991.

Terzakis JA: X-ray microanalysis. Problem solving in surgical pathology. *Path Annu* 20(pt 2):59–81, 1985.

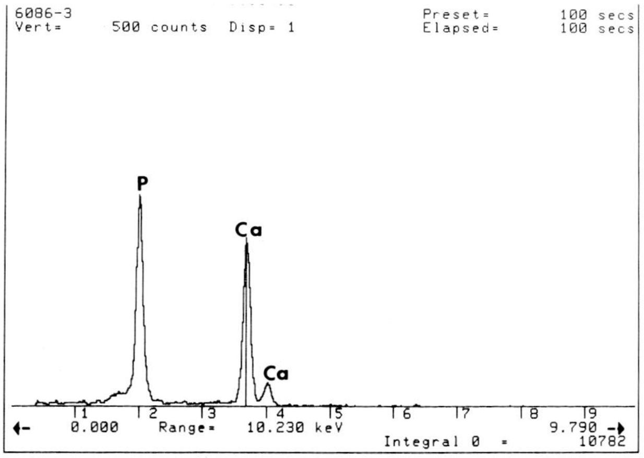

Fig. 8.22. Calcium pyrophosphate, EDX. The x-ray spectra of calcium pyrophosphate show equivalent P and Ca peaks.

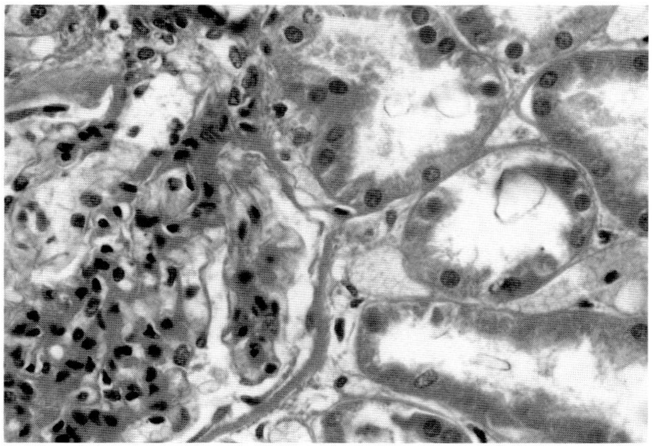

Fig. 8.23. Calcium oxalate, kidney. Renal tubules contain clear, irregular polygonal crystals of calcium oxalate.

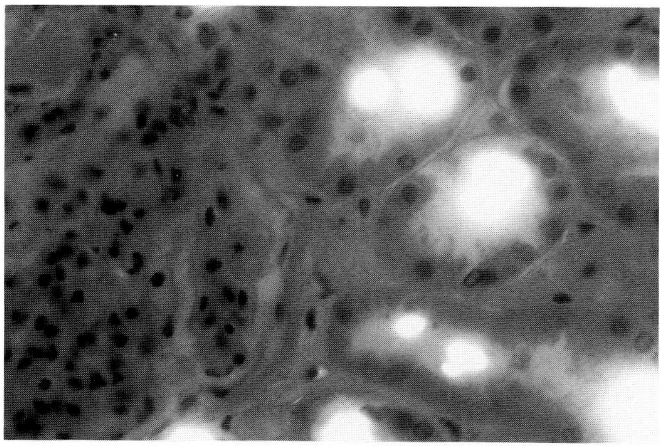

Fig. 8.24. Calcium oxalate, kidney, polarized light microscopy. Highly birefringent crystalline material is present in tubules, corresponding to Figure 8.23.

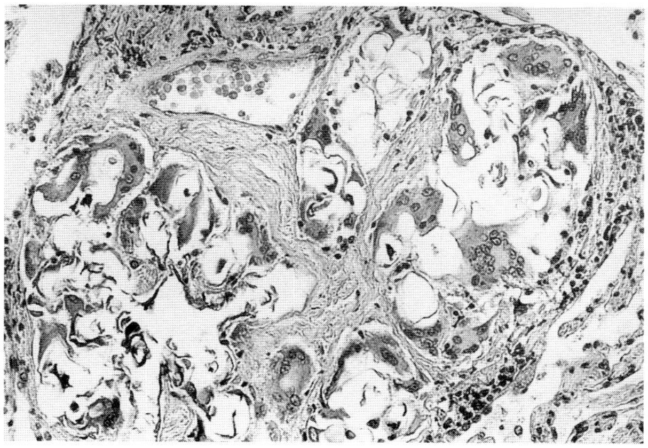

Fig. 8.25. Beryllium granuloma, lung. The granulomatous inflammation caused by beryllium contains black round particles and resembles those seen in sarcoidosis. However, atomic absorption spectroscopy or electron energy-loss spectroscopy will definitively identify beryllium.

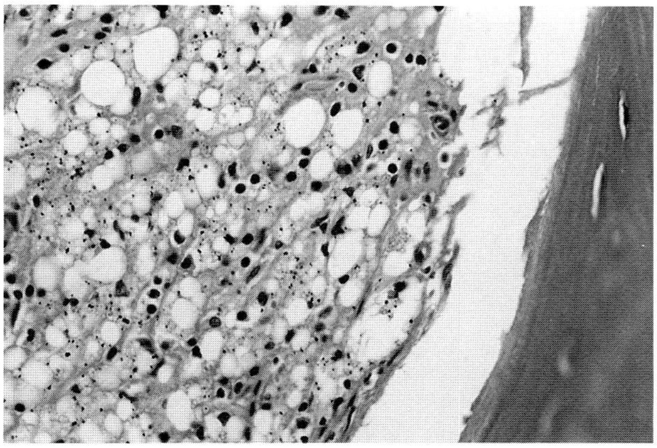

Fig. 8.26. Gold particles, bone. Gold particles are seen in the bone marrow of a patient treated with gold salts. The opaque gold particles can be seen in the cytoplasm of macrophages and in connective tissue, but they are not associated with a granulomatous reaction.

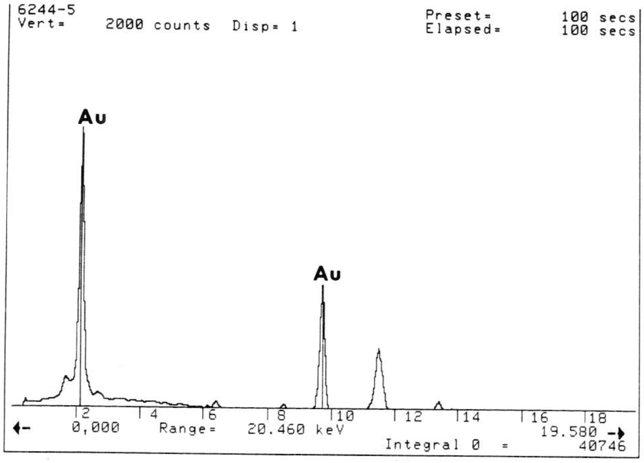

Fig. 8.27. Gold, energy-dispersive x-ray analysis. The typical gold signal of the previous biopsy is seen in this graph (Au peaks).

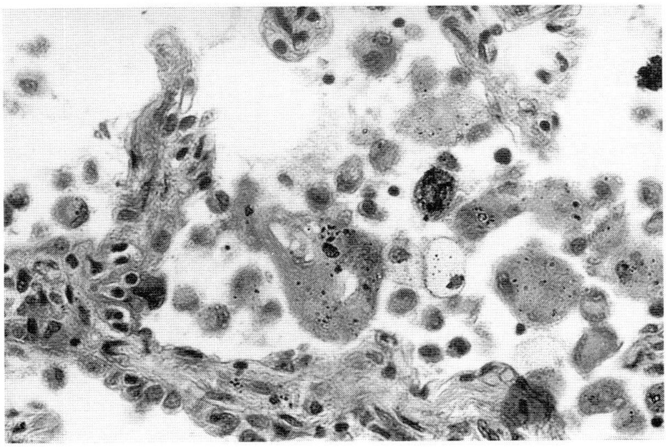

Fig. 8.28. Tungsten, lung. Black particles are seen in macrophages and giant cells.

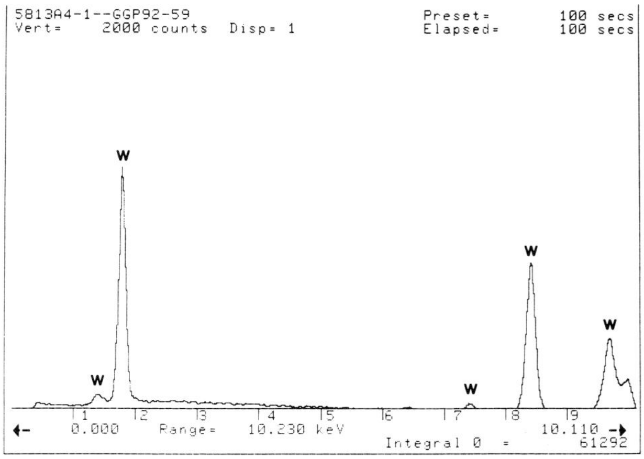

Fig. 8.29. Tungsten, EDX. The EDX of the previous specimen reveals characteristic peaks of tungsten.

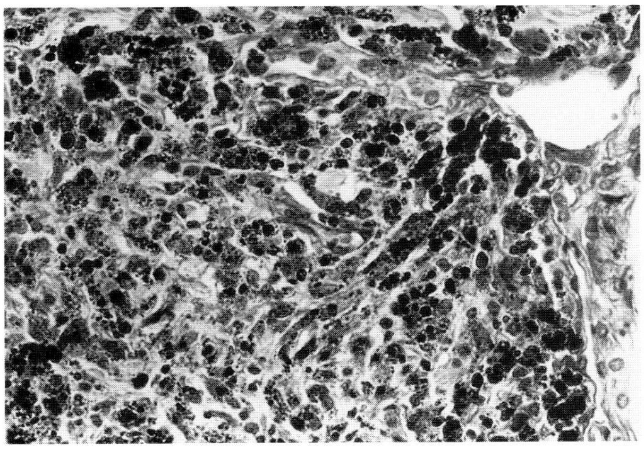

Fig. 8.30. Magnetite, lung. Interstitial deposits of iron are seen in the lung of an arc welder.

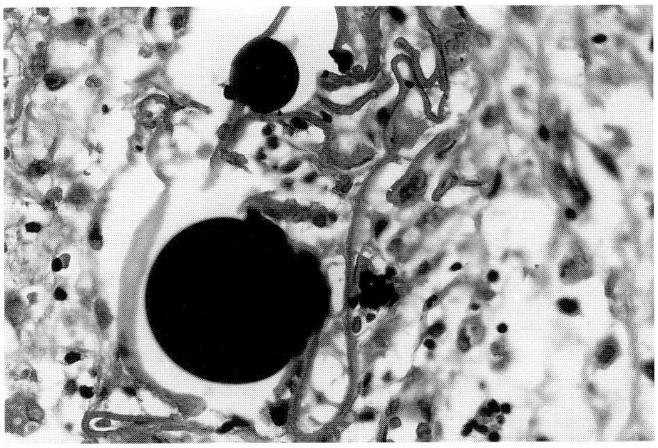

Fig. 8.31. Mercury granuloma. This patient suffered a traumatic injury from mercury-containing glass thermometer. Note the large black globules of evenly staining material.

Index

Note: Page numbers in italics refer to figures; page numbers followed by t refer to tables.

[redacted]